THE 4-WEEK
— FAST —
METABOLISM
Diet Plan

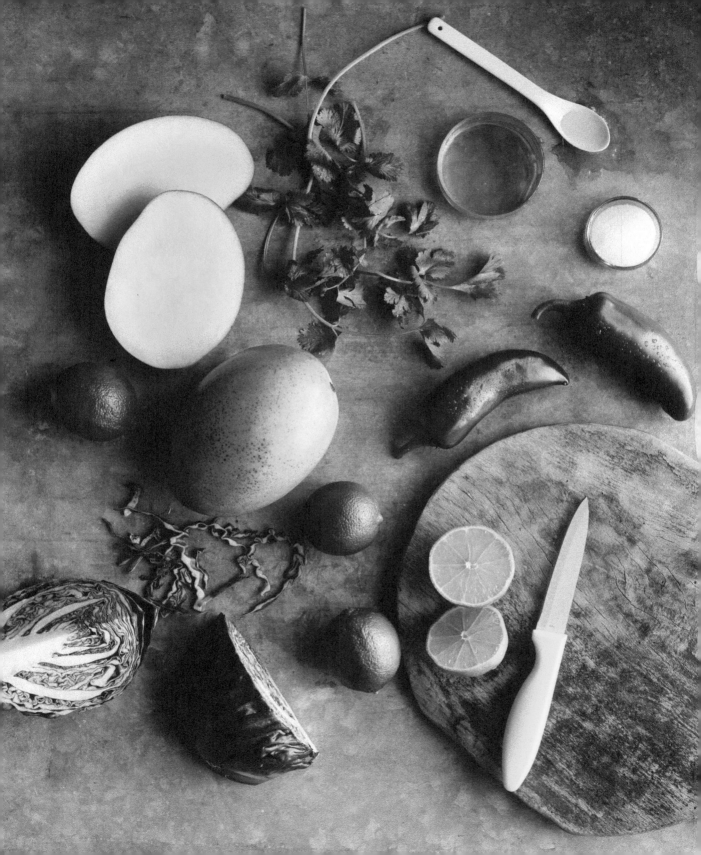

THE 4-WEEK
— FAST —
METABOLISM
Diet Plan

100 Recipes to
Reset Your Metabolism and Lose Weight

APRIL MURRAY, RD AND LEILA PAGE, RD

**ROCKRIDGE
PRESS**

For general information on our other products and services or to obtain technical support, please contact our Customer Care Department within the United States at (866) 744-2665, or outside the United States at (510) 253-0500.

Rockridge Press publishes its books in a variety of electronic and print formats. Some content that appears in print may not be available in electronic books, and vice versa.

Interior and Cover Designer: Lisa Forde
Art Producer: Hillary Frileck
Editor: Shannon Criss
Production Editor: Jenna Dutton

Photography ©2019 Elysa Weitala
Food styling by Victoria Wollard
Author photo courtesy of ©April Murray/Leila Page

ISBN: Print   978-1-64611-009-4
        eBook 978-1-64611-010-0

R0

We dedicate this book to our clients,
whose successes have fueled our desire
to continue helping others.

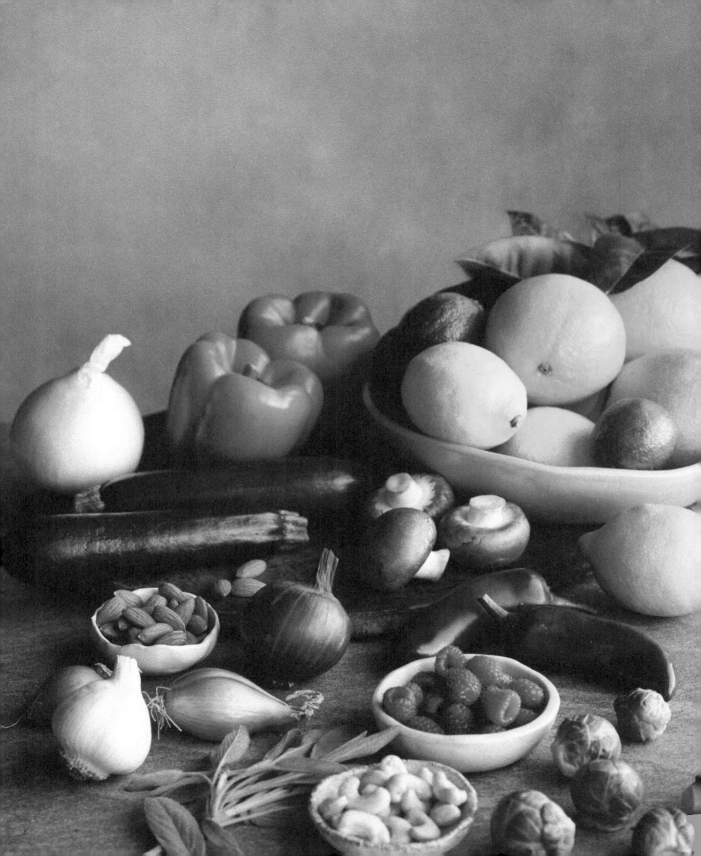

CONTENTS

INTRODUCTION

We want to start out by thanking you for picking up *The 4-Week Fast Metabolism Diet Plan*. We commend you for taking the time to invest in your health and choosing this book to assist you on your journey. Maybe you're feeling stuck at the moment. Maybe you have tried a handful of diets but haven't seen or felt any changes. Maybe you've been struggling with high blood sugar, weight gain, or low energy levels. We understand that life gets busy and that work commitments and packed schedules can often get in the way of your health. Trust us when we say we can help! We're committed to providing you with the best recipes, lifestyle tips, and evidence-based nutritional information out there.

We wrote this book based not only on our work as registered dietitians, but our personal experiences, too. As a young adult, April began to experience sudden weight gain and low energy levels. Without understanding exactly what was going on, she began restricting her calorie intake and working out more rigorously to shed the pounds. To her surprise, her weight continued to increase, and her energy levels became so low that she required more than 10 hours of sleep per day. Eventually along her health journey, she learned how the thyroid, adrenals, and metabolism functioned in relation to her symptoms. April then began working out less intensely and eating more nutrient-dense foods. Within months, her weight was within normal range and she felt like herself again.

Leila worked with a middle-aged woman struggling with a slow metabolism and an inability to lose weight. She had tried and failed at several diets, all of which left her feeling hungrier. After only a few months of eating clean, balanced meals, she lost 15 pounds. Another young woman came in wanting to lose weight for her wedding. She had been restricting her calories to less than 1,200 per day but was unsuccessful at losing the last 10 pounds. After two months of following a healthy meal plan, she lost the weight and felt energized for her wedding day!

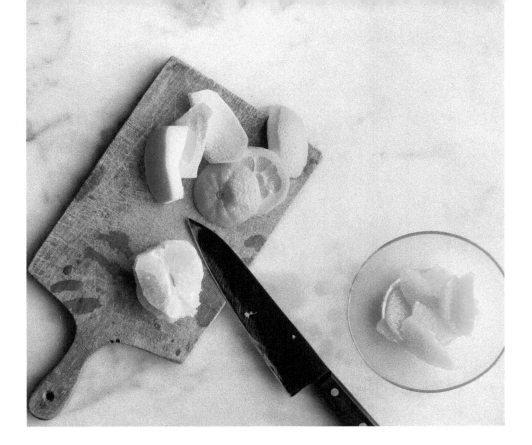

In our experience of working with a huge variety of individuals, we find that speeding up your metabolism is absolutely possible!

In this book, we explain why your metabolism may have slowed down and offer ways to reset your diet. We discuss the dos and don'ts when it comes to exercise, supplements, meal timing, sleeping habits, and much more. We hand-picked every single ingredient in this book based on its ability to affect your metabolism in a rewarding way. You will gain a new appreciation of your body and what you put into it.

We recommend starting our program when you can dedicate a solid four weeks to the plan without any special events or stressful work deadlines in the way. It can be challenging to turn down appetizers, cocktails, and desserts when you're on the road or vacationing.

Our passion is helping people feel and look better through manageable diet and lifestyle changes. We will be here to guide you through the kitchen, share our favorite recipes, and provide healthy lifestyle tips along the way. We are excited to help you feel like yourself again!

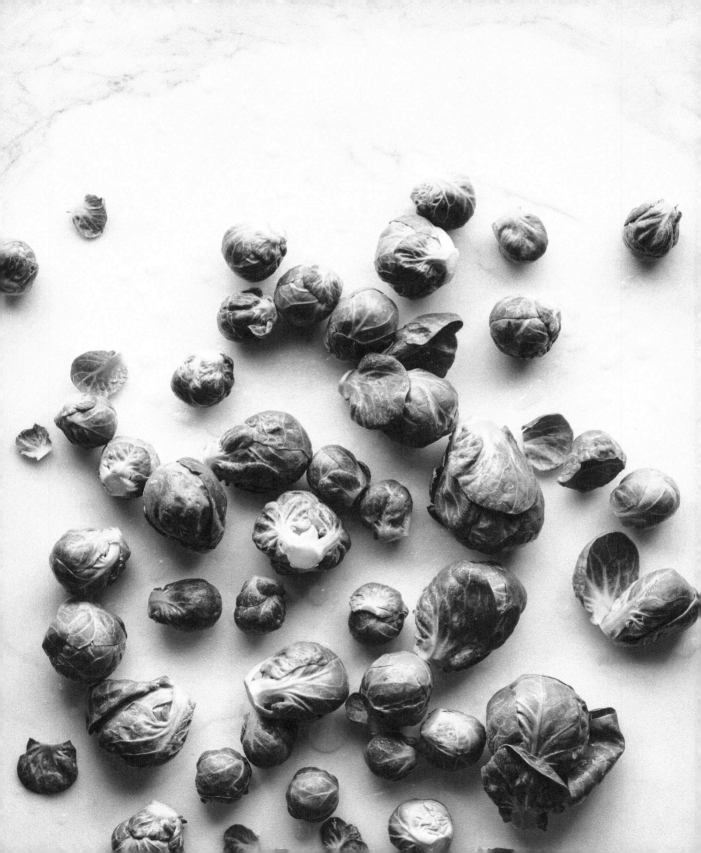

PART ONE

FAST METABOLISM 101

In this section, we will explain how *The 4-Week Fast Metabolism Diet Plan* can help you lose weight and feel more energized. You will learn why your metabolism plays such a big role in your overall health and well-being. We will also provide you with diet, exercise, and lifestyle tips so that you can speed up your metabolic rate. You will learn how to start losing fat and sustain your goals.

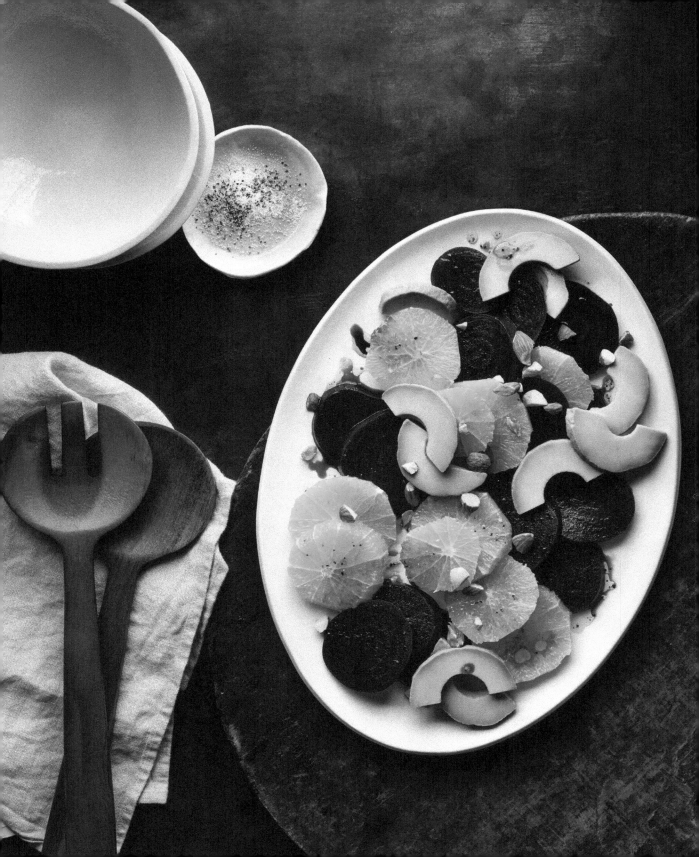

CHAPTER 1

Fast Metabolism Diet Basics

As dietitians in private practice, we meet with hundreds of individuals with the same goal of weight loss. Clients typically come to us because nothing seems to work for them anymore, not even the strictest fad diets or the most extreme exercise regimens. During our sessions, we have found that a slow metabolism is the common problem. Fortunately, for all of us, it is possible to accelerate our metabolism. In this chapter, we discuss modifiable lifestyle factors, such as diet, exercise, sleep, and meal timing that affect how many calories you burn per day.

ROASTED BEET CITRUS SALAD, PAGE 123

Understanding Your Metabolism

Through the process of metabolism, your body turns everything that you eat and drink into the energy it needs to survive. Even when you're asleep, your body needs energy for all of its hidden functions, such as breathing, circulating blood, and maintaining body temperature. On top of that, you burn calories when you do any physical activity—work out, complete house chores, and digest food, to name a few.

Let's take a look at what having a fast versus a slow metabolism looks and feels like. We all have that friend who doesn't eat perfectly but still maintains a fast metabolism. They are fit, energetic, and healthy. It doesn't seem fair, right? You might be reading this book because you are currently dealing with a sluggish metabolism. Maybe you have a very difficult time losing weight or feel as if you gain weight overnight. Working out doesn't seem to move the scale and you feel like you have to eat perfectly just to maintain your weight. Well, luckily for you, our book is designed to reset your metabolic rate—in only four weeks—using realistic diet and lifestyle changes. Not only will you lose weight, but you will feel better!

METABOLISM MYTHS

Extreme exercise can help me lose weight.

In most cases, over-exercising can actually do the opposite and slow down your weight-loss attempts. Excessive exercise puts stress on the body and typically makes you feel more hungry.

Thinner people have faster metabolisms.

Being thin doesn't mean that you're healthy. Have you heard the term "skinny-fat"? Well, it's a real thing. Some thin individuals lack substantial muscle mass and have high body fat percentages, meaning they have a slower metabolism.

As you age, your metabolism slows down.

Your muscle mass declines as you get older if you're not careful! Fortunately, weight-bearing exercises can prevent muscle loss, keeping your metabolism steady.

I was born with a slow metabolism and there's nothing I can do to change it.

Genetics play only a small role in your total metabolic rate.

Eating a very low-calorie diet is a great weight loss solution.

Eating too few calories slows down your metabolism.

The Fast Metabolism Diet and Exercise Connection

There are three main components associated with resetting your metabolism. All of these factors influence your metabolism either directly or indirectly, because metabolism is affected by lifestyle and not just by heredity.

1. **Exercise:** Muscle-building exercises are key to boosting your metabolism. The more muscle you have, the faster your metabolism will be! We recommend moderate exercise over extreme exercise. Even 15-minute stints will help preserve and activate your muscles. Lean muscle is active tissue, meaning it burns calories even while you are asleep. Pairing exercise with *The 4-Week Fast Metabolism Diet Plan* will give you better results.

2. **Diet:** Eat adequate amounts of high-quality protein, fiber, vitamins, minerals, and phytonutrients throughout the day.

3. **Sleep:** Your body is best able to burn stored fat during prolonged, deep sleep. Aim for at least seven to nine hours of sleep each night. Good-quality sleep also prevents your body from releasing excess cortisol, a hormone that blocks fat loss.

Here are 10 foods that are known to boost your metabolism. The recipes in this book will include delicious ways to incorporate these foods into your diet.

Beets: contain compounds that help detoxify the liver and other digestive organs, which are important for weight loss.

Grass-fed beef: compared to conventionally raised beef, grass-fed typically contains fewer calories, more omega-3 fatty acids, and higher amounts of vitamins A and E.

Chia seeds: a great source of fiber, omega-3 fatty acids, potassium, magnesium, and protein—all of which are important for our metabolism.

Cruciferous vegetables: contain B vitamins, vitamin C, calcium, and fiber. Vegetables such as broccoli, cauliflower, and cabbage are nutritionally dense with very few calories.

Eggs: the yolks are rich in a wide array of vitamins and minerals.

Berries: studies have shown their potential metabolism-boosting effects due to the presence of anthocyanin compounds.

Salmon: fatty fish such as salmon helps your liver during detoxification and provides your body with protein.

Spinach: extremely high in iron, a mineral that helps carry the oxygen your muscles need to burn fat.

Legumes: beans, peas, and lentils are a perfect way to get quality dietary protein and fiber, both of which help create a feeling of fullness and keep blood sugar within a healthy range.

Flaxseed meal: in addition to containing omega-3 fats, flaxseeds are an excellent source of fiber and lignans, a phytonutrient that helps prevent insulin resistance.

OTHER FACTORS THAT AFFECT METABOLISM

Muscle mass: Luckily, muscle mass is a component of your metabolism that you can control. When you increase your muscle mass, you boost your metabolic rate, meaning you burn more calories. By doing weight training, getting enough rest, and eating adequate amounts of protein, you can boost your muscle mass.

Age: As we all know, you cannot alter your age. But on the bright side, the main reason your metabolism slows down as you age is loss of muscle mass—which you *can* control!

Body size: The more you weigh, the more calories you tend to burn. Think about it: It takes a lot more effort for a six-foot-eight man to run one mile than a five-foot-one woman. As you lose weight, especially if you're losing muscle, your metabolism and weight loss begin to slow down.

Gender: Women get the worse part of the deal when it comes to metabolism. In general, men tend to burn more calories than women due to higher testosterone levels and, therefore, more lean muscle mass.

Hormones: Your hormone levels are affected by your diet, sleep, exercise, stress levels, and more. Keeping hormones such as insulin, ghrelin, and cortisol within normal range supports weight loss.

Environment: By lowering your toxic burden, you free up your liver's ability to metabolize fat, rather than spending time detoxifying harmful substances from your body.

Drugs: A healthy diet and lifestyle can help minimize your chances of needing to take medication. For many, however, medication is crucial to health. Some medications can make you feel hungrier while others slow your body's ability to burn calories or cause you to hold on to extra fluids.

Genetics: Emerging research has shown that you can turn certain genes on and off by living a healthy lifestyle.

Living the Fast Metabolism Lifestyle

Here are the three pillars of our fast metabolism lifestyle. Remember that it's important to incorporate all three into your day-to-day life for the best results. For instance, a perfect diet and exercise routine won't make up for a lack of sleep.

Mealtimes: Part of resetting your metabolism involves regulating your blood sugar levels. The average meal should provide three to four hours of stable energy and blood sugar. We encourage eating at least three balanced meals per day, plus a few snacks. You should eat your first meal of the day within one hour of waking up. We also recommend a 12-hour overnight fasting window to allow your body to rest and repair.

Exercise: On the metabolism reset plan, we recommend moderate amounts of exercise with a focus on preserving lean muscle mass. The program may take longer to work if you skip the exercises entirely or exercise more than recommended. The best time to exercise is in the morning or during the day. If possible, avoid exercising late in the evening, as this can disrupt sleep for some people. Another great way to fit in exercise during the day is by taking the stairs at work or parking farther away from the store to get in more steps. Our program involves walking seven days a week for 30 minutes, doing body-weight exercise four days a week for 15 minutes, and engaging in one exercise of choice per week.

Rest and recovery: Many experts believe that sleep affects your weight more than diet or exercise. When you don't get enough sleep, your hunger and fullness hormones are greatly affected. You tend to feel hungrier and crave more carbohydrates and sweets when you are not well rested. This is one of the reasons why we would like you to avoid caffeine on our program.

Curcumin: For centuries, curcumin (a component of turmeric) has been thought to have anti-inflammatory qualities, which may help with weight loss. Black pepper has been shown to activate curcumin in the body.

Milk thistle: Milk thistle acts as an antioxidant, lowers liver inflammation, reduces triglycerides within the liver, improves insulin sensitivity, and helps you burn fuel more efficiently. It can be taken in food form (milk thistle seeds must be blended or ground) or as a supplement.

Reishi: Reishi mushrooms can help balance hormone levels and keep blood sugar stable. These mushrooms are edible and mostly found as supplements in the form of capsules and powders.

Resveratrol: This popular phytonutrient has made its way into the news for its ability to promote a healthy aging process by reducing inflammation and blood sugar levels. Food sources of resveratrol include grapes.

Catechins: Catechins are one of the bitter compounds found in green tea. Green tea has been shown to reduce blood pressure and blood fats, and may even help lower blood sugar.

Before starting any supplement, you should always check with your health care practitioner.

THE FAST METABOLISM DIET RULES

There are eight fast metabolism rules you must follow to reap the most benefits from the diet.

1. **Avoid alcohol.** It dehydrates the body, raises blood sugar levels, and contributes to chronic inflammation.

2. **Eat enough protein.** Your body burns more calories digesting protein than other macronutrients, which is why you should include some form of protein in every meal.

3. **Strive for seven to nine hours of sleep per night.** Several studies note that inadequate sleep may lower your metabolic rate and increase your likelihood of weight gain.

4. **Avoid caffeine.** Caffeine increases cortisol, a stress hormone that causes fat to be stored around the abdomen.

5. **Follow the exercise protocol.** Regular resistance training exercises are key to building muscle. Muscle is harder to build and maintain as you age. Most of us start losing muscle around age 30, with a 3 percent to 8 percent reduction in lean muscle mass every decade thereafter.

6. **Drink enough water.** Proper hydration helps grease the wheels of your digestive system, encouraging food to be metabolized more quickly. To determine your needs, measure your body weight in pounds and divide in half. The result is the number of ounces of water you should drink each day.

7. **Buy clean and organic foods.** Our plan emphasizes reducing your intake of toxins by encouraging the intake of organically grown, non–genetically modified foods; lean, grass-fed animal meats; and wild-caught fish. We strongly encourage you to use these clean ingredients for all the recipes in this book.

8. **Eat enough to fuel your body.** Lowering your calorie intake can ultimately decrease your metabolic rate as the body tries to conserve energy. To keep energy levels high and your metabolism engaged, it's important to not to restrict calories too much or else you could put your body into starvation mode. The goal is to make sure you're eating enough but also to avoid feeling overly full.

Fruit juice: Drinking fruit juice (including fresh-squeezed) can wreak havoc on your metabolism in several ways, including causing sluggishness, food cravings, and inflammation. If you are craving juice, choose a green juice that is completely vegetable-based (e.g., carrot-ginger-spinach).

"Healthy" packaged foods: Don't let the packaging fool you; always check the ingredients list before you buy. Chips, crackers, pretzels, and, yes, even gluten-free cookies typically contain empty calories. Avoid packaged foods that contain processed vegetable oils such as corn and soy, as these are high in omega-6 fats (polyunsaturated fats that, when eaten in excess, can lead to inflammatory conditions such as heart disease). A good basic rule is to make sure the food contains fewer than 3 grams of sugar per 100 calories.

White flour: It absorbs rapidly into your bloodstream, meaning if you don't burn it, you're going to store white flour as fat.

Refined sugars: Research has shown that calories derived from sugar are more easily converted into belly fat compared to calories from protein, fat, or vegetables.

Artificial sweeteners: Artificial sweeteners include sucralose (knows as Splenda), sugar alcohols such as xylitol, and highly processed sugars such as high-fructose corn syrup. In comparison to honey or maple syrup, artificial sweeteners tend to be much sweeter in flavor. We want you to train your taste buds to think a fresh peach has the perfect sweetness.

The 4-Week Fast Metabolism Diet Plan aims to make your metabolism faster, so you burn fat instead of storing it. Before you begin this four-week program, remember that one to two pounds per week is considered a healthy rate of weight loss. People who lose weight gradually are more successful at keeping the weight off. The more body fat you have to lose, the more dramatic your results will be. Those of you with less weight to lose will see less significant results.

Because you are cutting sugar, alcohol, and caffeine out of your diet, expect to feel a little more sluggish and "hangry" the first few days. But don't worry, after your first full week on the diet, you can expect to feel more energized than when you started! After two to three weeks, you will find that the diet gets easier and will start to become more of a lifestyle. Once you've completed the four-week plan and notice success with weight loss, you may find yourself wanting to continue the program. And with a faster metabolism, you will find it easier to maintain your weight loss.

If you hit a weight-loss plateau, understand that this is totally normal. Weight loss is a stressor on the body and shouldn't be rushed. When losing significant amounts of weight, plan to carve out a few weeks at a time to focus on maintaining the weight you have lost so far. This leads to better long-term weight loss success.

Planning Ahead and Cooking Efficiently

When cooking at home, the key to being successful is planning ahead and cooking efficiently. Here are some handy hacks for time management in the kitchen:

» Choose one day out of the week to get your shopping done. Bring a grocery list and be sure to buy all your ingredients for that week.

» Choose frozen precooked grains to cut down on cooking time. Most markets now carry frozen cooked brown rice and quinoa. These items take only a few minutes to heat up in the microwave and are a healthy, fast option to speed up total cooking time.

» Prepare the item that takes the longest amount of time to cook first. In most meals, there are different components that make up the meal, such as a protein, carbohydrates, and vegetables. By starting on the component that takes the longest, such as brown rice, and then preparing the rest while that is cooking, you can make sure the meal gets cooked in a reasonable amount of time.

» Check your supermarket produce aisles for pre-chopped fresh vegetables. If time is more of a concern than money, then buying these pre-prepped vegetables can be a valuable time-saver. However, they will go bad sooner than whole vegetables, so use them earlier in the week.

» Order groceries online for delivery when you are very busy. Buying groceries online can save an abundance of time and alleviate the stress of a hectic to-do list.

STORAGE HACKS

Here are some storage hacks that will keep your foods safe and save you time:

» When preparing a meal, store leftover chopped vegetables in a glass storage container for later use. This will save you money and time for the next recipe.

» Place leftovers in individual glass containers to take with you to work the next day. This will help you save time preparing lunch the next morning.

» Glass containers are safest when it comes to reheating foods and best for the environment. We choose glass containers over plastic because many plastic containers have harmful BPA compounds that can be absorbed as toxins by your body.

About the Recipes

Each of our metabolism-boosting recipes is labeled to guide you through this journey. Working in private practice, we're familiar with the busy routine of the average individual. The thought of cooking a meal can be overwhelming, leading many of us to order delivery or stop for fast food. We don't have to tell you that eating out wreaks havoc on your metabolism, as you probably already know or have experienced yourself. We developed these recipes with your busy schedule in mind. We know that you (and your family) will love them; we sure do!

As you glance through the recipes, you will see that many can be prepared in 30 minutes or less and use just a handful of ingredients. All the ingredients can easily be found at your local market. Another time saver is the Complete Meal recipes. You won't have to worry about preparing side dishes to pair with these.

We've included recipe options for vegan and vegetarian diets to reset your metabolism. For individuals with digestive issues or lactose-intolerance, use only the dairy-free recipes. Most of our recipes are gluten-free—ideal for individuals with gluten sensitivity, celiac disease, or other autoimmune conditions.

All herbs and spices are allowed in the meal plan, but some offer targeted health benefits related to metabolism.

Ginger: stimulates digestion, circulation, and sweating—processes that help cleanse the colon, liver, and other detox organs.

Turmeric: known for its liver-detoxifying properties, as well as its anti-inflammatory and cancer-fighting characteristics. Absorption of curcumin, a component of turmeric, is increased by black pepper, so turmeric and black pepper should be eaten together.

Himalayan salt: occurs naturally and is not chemically processed or refined. It also contains iron, magnesium, phosphorus, calcium, potassium, and chloride—nutrients helpful for metabolism functions.

Cayenne pepper: the active ingredient in cayenne pepper, known as capsaicin, increases the body temperature, which promotes calorie-burning.

Rosemary: enhances bile flow, which helps with fat metabolism and detoxification. This increases nutrient absorption and helps reduce the body's toxic load.

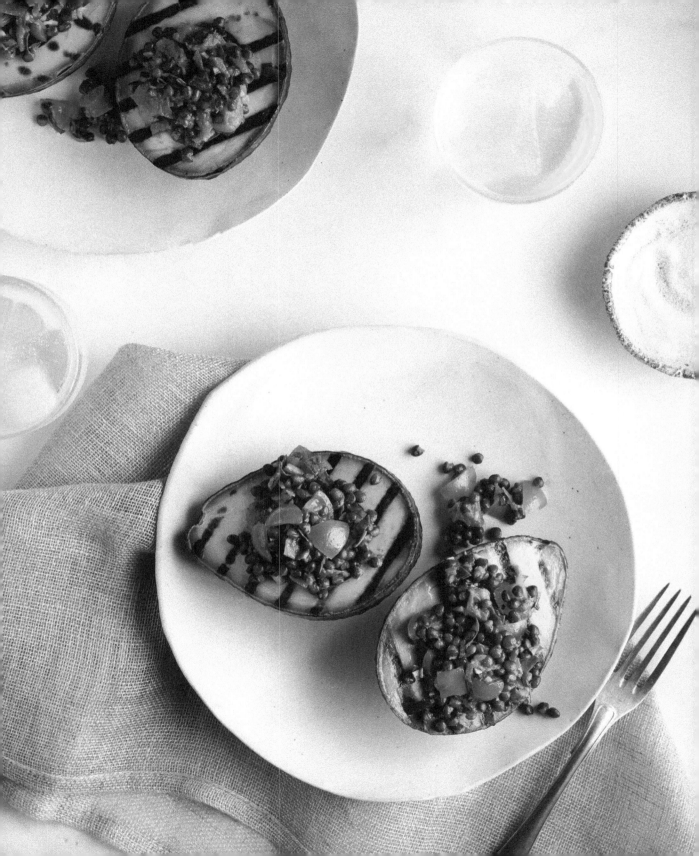

CHAPTER 2

The 4-Week Plan

It's time to get into the juicy details; we hope you're excited to get started! This chapter will provide you with everything you need to begin the plan and stick with it through the four weeks—and beyond.

The Meal Plan

» This meal plan is structured for two people and each recipe yields two or four servings. That means for the four-serving recipes, expect to have two servings of leftovers. The idea is that you can use the leftovers for lunch or dinner the next day.

» Each week includes a shopping list so you know exactly what you need to buy for the week. Take the shopping list with you to the grocery store (or snap a quick photo) and use it to do your weekly shopping.

» If the shopping list doesn't specify an exact amount (such as a 12-ounce jar of marinara sauce or 8 eggs), just buy a bottle/can/jar/bunch of the ingredient. This includes things like oil and salt and dried herbs. You will see them in the Week One Shopping List but not in the subsequent lists, because one purchase will last you several weeks.

» When the meal plan refers to a specific recipe that's in Part Two, we'll include the page number where you can find it.

» An asterisk next to a recipe in the meal plan means that it will be used for leftovers. You may choose to double the recipe if the yield isn't enough for your family or if you don't think you will have enough food for leftovers.

» Every week, we will offer two meal substitution suggestions, in case you prefer a different recipe or flavor profile.

» During the four weeks, we recommend eating both snacks to stabilize blood sugar levels in between meals.

» Variety is key for overall health. We do not recommend eating the same breakfast or snack every day. Do your best to follow the meal plan as it is laid out.

» Non-starchy vegetables such as cucumbers, bell peppers, and jicama are considered free foods, meaning you can eat as much as you'd like. Feel free to snack on these throughout the day or add them to a meal to bulk up the portion size.

» We recommend eating no more than three desserts per week. Chapter 7 has lots of healthy dessert recipes. You can also enjoy any fruit you like or decaf tea to diminish cravings for sweets.

» Not all the recipes in this book are included in the four-week meal plan, so you will have lots of recipes to choose from even after you complete the reset phase.

The Exercise Plan

In the four-week exercise plan, we introduce an easy and effective way to support your fast metabolism journey. Exercise will not only help you lose weight but *maintain* your ideal weight.

You may be surprised to find that these exercises are low intensity. This is intentional. Excessive exercise and over-training often slow down weight-loss efforts. Remember that exercise is a stressor on the body (it releases cortisol and adrenaline hormones), so if you're already sleep-deprived and stressed out, it's better to opt for lighter workouts. Intensive exercise also causes excessive hunger, which can make it difficult to maintain a calorie deficit and lose weight.

In our practice, clients often see better results when they follow a lighter exercise regimen such as walking, yoga, light weight training, and, yes, even rest days! After the four weeks, feel free to reintroduce your previous workouts back into your routine.

This four-week plan will provide a practical and obtainable method to increase your metabolism, as well as maintain a healthy weight and lifestyle. To succeed with weight loss, calories out need to outweigh calories in. To maintain your weight, you need to balance calories in and out. Achieving this includes exercising to burn calories. Not only will exercise burn calories, but it will also reduce your risk of heart disease, improve your mood, and help manage insulin levels, in addition to numerous other health benefits.

Building muscle to boost your metabolism is one of the many rewards of exercise. As we mentioned in chapter 1, building muscle is an important factor in improving your resting metabolic rate. By increasing lean muscle tissue, your body is able to burn more calories. For every pound of muscle, your body burns about six calories at rest per day. (In contrast, a pound of fat burns about two calories.) So if you were to gain five pounds of muscle, you would burn an extra 20 calories a day. Over a year, you would burn an extra 7,300 calories—by doing nothing! With this in mind, our exercise plan will gradually help you gain muscle mass so you can burn more calories.

The exercise plan consists of four workout days, two days of rest, and one day for personal choice. In addition to strength training exercises, you will be incorporating walks into your day. Specifically, the routine will focus on cardio and body-weight strength training (organized by core, upper body, lower body, and full body). Each day consists of four exercises that should take 30 minutes to complete. The exercises will increase slightly in difficulty every week. During week four, you will revisit the exercises in week one to keep your body and you from getting physically or mentally burnt out. Redoing week-one exercises will give you the opportunity to see how far you've come in terms of your strength and energy levels. The exercise routines can be completed at home with little to no equipment, but there will be options for treadmill exercise, if you have one.

Week One

We are so excited for you! You're starting week one of our fast metabolism plan. During the first seven days, expect to go through an adjustment period as you'll be trying some new foods and recipes. You'll learn to incorporate a wide variety of proteins, vegetables, and spices into your diet, including pork tenderloin, beets, and turmeric. Don't be surprised if the Ground Turkey Tacos with Tropical Mango Slaw become your new weeknight go-to meal.

WEEK ONE SHOPPING LIST

CANNED, BOTTLED, AND JARRED ITEMS

- Almond butter
- Avocado oil
- Artichoke hearts, 1 (12-ounce) jar
- Balsamic vinegar
- Coconut aminos
- Coconut milk, light (1 cup)
- Honey
- Marinara sauce, 1 (12-ounce) jar (less than 260 mg of sodium per serving)
- Olive oil, extra-virgin
- Olive tapenade (¼ cup)
- Red wine vinegar
- Vanilla extract, pure

DAIRY AND EGGS

- Eggs (17)
- Goat cheese (7 ounces)
- Greek yogurt, plain low-fat, 1 (40-ounce) container
- Parmesan cheese, shredded (¼ cup)

MEAT, POULTRY, AND SEAFOOD

- Canadian bacon, nitrate-free, 4 slices
- Chicken breasts, 4 boneless, skinless
- Chicken tenders (1 pound)
- Grass-fed flank steak (1 pound)
- Pork tenderloin (1 pound)
- Shrimp, jumbo, 24 unpeeled raw (about 2 pounds)
- Turkey, lean ground (1 pound)

PANTRY ITEMS

- Almonds, unsalted (1¼ cups)
- Brown sugar
- Chia seeds (2 tablespoons, includes snacks)
- Chili powder
- Coffee, ground
- Cornstarch
- Cumin, ground

- English muffins, whole-wheat (1 package)
- Farro, uncooked (1 cup)
- Garlic powder
- Ginger, ground
- Onion powder
- Oregano, dried
- Panko (Japanese large breadcrumbs), whole-wheat
- Paprika, smoked
- Pepper
- Red pepper flakes
- Rice (brown, jasmine, basmati, or short grain), uncooked (1 cup)
- Rosemary, dried
- Salt
- Sourdough bread
- Turmeric, ground

PRODUCE

- Arugula (4 cups)
- Avocado (1)
- Beets (4)
- Beets, small (8)
- Bell peppers, red (3)
- Broccoli (1 bunch)
- Brussels sprouts (1 pound)
- Cabbage, purple (4 cups)
- English cucumber (1 large)
- Fennel (1 bulb)
- Garlic (2 heads)
- Ginger, fresh, 1 (3-inch) piece
- Jalapeño pepper (1)
- Lemons (6)
- Limes (3)
- Mangos, small (3)
- Onions, yellow (2 medium)
- Oranges (2)
- Papaya, small (1)
- Shallot (1)
- Spinach, fresh (1 cup)
- Zucchini noodles (fresh or frozen), 2 packages store-bought

FRESH HERBS

- Cilantro, fresh
- Dill, fresh
- Oregano, fresh
- Thyme, fresh

WEEK 1: MEAL PLAN

Meal substitutions:

» Veggie Fried Rice (page 65) for Beet and Goat Cheese Frittata with Arugula Salad (page 68)

» Sesame-Crusted Salmon (page 83) for Beef Stir-Fry (page 112)

MONDAY

BREAKFAST	Balanced Breakfast Sandwich (page 59)
LUNCH	Mediterranean Farro Salad (page 137)
DINNER	Greek Lemony Oregano Chicken* (page 99) + Roasted Beet Citrus Salad* (page 123)
SNACK 1	1 cup low-fat plain Greek yogurt + 1 tablespoon almonds
SNACK 2	3 tablespoons crumbled goat cheese + 1 cup sliced bell peppers

TUESDAY

BREAKFAST	Papaya Greek Yogurt Bowl (page 53)
LUNCH	Leftovers: Greek Lemony Oregano Chicken + Roasted Beet Citrus Salad
DINNER	Garlicky Shrimp Scampi* (page 91) + 1 slice sourdough bread
SNACK 1	1 hardboiled egg
SNACK 2	1 cup sliced mango

WEDNESDAY

BREAKFAST	Balanced Breakfast Sandwich (page 59)
LUNCH	Leftovers: Garlicky Shrimp Scampi + 1 slice sourdough bread
DINNER	Ground Turkey Tacos* (page 107) + Tropical Mango Slaw* (page 121)
SNACK 1	3 tablespoons crumbled goat cheese + 1 cup sliced bell peppers
SNACK 2	3 tablespoons almonds

THURSDAY

BREAKFAST	Papaya Greek Yogurt Bowl (*page 53*)
LUNCH	Leftovers: Ground Turkey Tacos + Tropical Mango Slaw
DINNER	Beef Stir-Fry* (*page 112*) + Coconut Brown Rice* (*page 135*)
SNACK 1	3 tablespoons crumbled goat cheese + 1 cup sliced bell peppers
SNACK 2	1 hardboiled egg

FRIDAY

BREAKFAST	Balanced Breakfast Sandwich (*page 59*)
LUNCH	Leftovers: Beef Stir-Fry + Coconut Brown Rice
DINNER	Coffee-Rubbed Pork Tenderloin* (*page 109*) + Crispy Roasted Brussels Sprouts with Balsamic Drizzle* (*page 125*)
SNACK 1	3 tablespoons almonds
SNACK 2	½ cup plain low-fat Greek yogurt + 1 tablespoon almonds

SATURDAY

BRUNCH	Beet and Goat Cheese Frittata with Arugula Salad (*page 68*)
DINNER	Leftovers: Coffee-Rubbed Pork Tenderloin + Crispy Roasted Brussels Sprouts with Balsamic Drizzle
SNACK 1	1 hardboiled egg
SNACK 2	1 whole-wheat English muffin + 1 tablespoon almond butter

SUNDAY

BRUNCH	Artichoke Turmeric Shakshuka (*page 66*)
DINNER	Crispy Parmesan Rosemary Chicken Tenders* (*page 102*) + Zesty Broccoli with Garlic and Red Pepper Flakes* (*page 124*)
SNACK 1	1 cup low-fat plain Greek yogurt + 1 tablespoon chia seeds
SNACK 2	1 cup sliced mango + 3 tablespoons almonds

WEEK ONE EXERCISE PLAN

You will begin with light exercises that will ease your body into building muscle. No equipment is required. Complete one set of the core, upper body, lower body, and full body exercises, then take a break for water, and repeat for a total of two sets. Finish with some stretching of your choice and remember to include a walk at some point in your day. If you have a difficult time doing a particular exercise, simply double up on a different exercise you feel more comfortable with.

Core: *Plank—Position your body similar to a push-up, but resting on your forearms, which should be about shoulder-length apart on the ground. Hold for 30 seconds.*

Upper Body: *Arm Scissors—Stand with your legs shoulder-width apart and stretch your arms forward. Then move your arms out to the sides and in across your body, alternating the right and left arm on top as they cross in the middle. That's one repetition. Complete 10 for one set.*

Lower Body: *Forward Lunges—Stand with your legs together, then thrust one leg forward into a deep lunge. Come back to a standing position and repeat with the other leg. Complete 10 with each leg for one set.*

Full Body: *Burpees—Stand with your legs together and your arms down at your sides. Jump up and reach for the sky with your arms. Quickly transition to a push-up position and do one push-up. Jump back up and repeat. Complete 3 burpees for one set.*

Stretching: *After completing two sets of these four exercises, end your workout by stretching for 5 or more minutes.*

Cardio: *Walk—Take a briskly paced walk around the block or on a treadmill for 30 minutes. We suggest walking outside for some vitamin D.*

Week Two

If you are following this plan with hopes of losing weight, remember that weight loss occurs through a slight calorie deficit. Counting calories is not required; however, we do encourage you to tune in to your hunger and fullness cues. The goal is to eat just enough so that you're satisfied but not stuffed. Don't feel as if you need to finish everything on your plate. If you feel overly hungry this week, we encourage you to have an extra snack (see chapter 7 for snack ideas).

SHOPPING LIST

CANNED, BOTTLED, AND JARRED ITEMS

- Avocado mayonnaise (2 tablespoons)
- Avocado oil spray
- Capers
- Chicken stock, low-sodium (½ cup)
- Chickpeas, no-salt-added, 1 (15-ounce) can

- Coconut milk, unsweetened (1 cup)
- Green chilies, mild chopped, 2 (4-ounce) cans
- Mustard, grainy (2 tablespoons)
- Pomegranate juice (1 cup)

- Rice wine vinegar, seasoned (3 tablespoons)
- Sun-dried tomato pesto (¼ cup)
- Vegetable broth, low-sodium (2 cups)
- Worcestershire sauce

DAIRY AND EGGS

- Eggs (16)

- Milk, 1 percent (1 cup)

- Parmesan cheese, grated (¼ cup)

MEAT, POULTRY, AND SEAFOOD

- Chicken breasts, boneless, skinless (3½ pounds)
- Chicken tenders (1 pound)

- Lox (6 ounces)
- Pink salmon, skinless, boneless, canned (20 ounces)

- Pork tenderloin (1 pound)

PANTRY ITEMS

- Brown rice, uncooked (1 cup)
- Chia seeds (¼ cup)
- Cinnamon
- Everything bagels, whole-wheat (we like Ezekiel Bread) (3)
- Flaxseeds, ground (2 tablespoons)
- Hemp seeds, hulled (2 tablespoons)
- Lemon pepper
- Panko, whole-wheat
- Pita bread, whole-wheat (1 package)
- Quinoa, uncooked (1 cup)
- Rolled oats, whole-grain (1 cup)
- Walnuts (1½ cups)

PRODUCE

- Apples (2)
- Arugula (2 cups)
- Avocados, medium (3)
- Carrots, large (4)
- Cauliflower, large (1)
- Cherry tomatoes (1 pint)
- Corn (4 ears)
- English Cucumbers (3)
- Garlic (10 cloves)
- Jalapeño peppers (2)
- Lemons (3)
- Limes (2)
- Onion, red (1)
- Onion, Vidalia (or yellow onion), medium (1)
- Onion, white, small (1)
- Onions, yellow, medium (2)
- Potatoes, baby, multicolored (1 pound)
- Scallions (3)
- Shallot (1)
- Spinach (4 cups)
- Tomato (1)

FRESH HERBS

- Cilantro, fresh
- Dill, fresh
- Parsley, flat-leaf, fresh
- Sage, fresh
- Thyme, fresh

WEEK TWO MEAL PLAN

Meal substitutions:

» Apple Cinnamon Oatmeal (page 56) for Carrot Cake Overnight Oats with Flax and Walnuts

» Blackened Tilapia (page 77) for Salmon Cakes

MONDAY

BREAKFAST Carrot Cake Overnight Oats with Flax and Walnuts* *(page 55)*

LUNCH Leftovers from Week One: Crispy Parmesan Rosemary Chicken Tenders + Zesty Broccoli with Garlic and Red Pepper Flakes

DINNER Sun-Dried Tomato Roasted Chicken* *(page 101)* + Lemon Pepper Cauliflower Steaks Topped with Panko* *(page 126)*

SNACK 1 ½ avocado sprinkled with salt

SNACK 2 1 cup sliced cucumbers + 2 tablespoons tzatziki *(from Tzatziki Yogurt Sauce with Whole-Wheat Pita, page 145)*

TUESDAY

BREAKFAST Avocado and Lox Bagel *(page 58)*

LUNCH Leftovers: Sun-Dried Tomato Roasted Chicken + Lemon Pepper Cauliflower Steaks Topped with Panko

DINNER Salmon Cakes* *(page 84)* + Spanakopita Rice* *(page 136)* with tzatziki

SNACK 1 3 tablespoons walnuts

SNACK 2 1 cup carrots

WEDNESDAY

BREAKFAST Leftovers: Carrot Cake Overnight Oats with Flax and Walnuts

LUNCH Leftovers: Salmon Cakes + Spanakopita Rice with tzatziki

DINNER Green Chili Baked Chicken* *(page 97)* + Lime Quinoa* *(page 134)*

SNACK 1 1 apple

SNACK 2 1 hardboiled egg

THURSDAY

BREAKFAST .... Avocado and Lox Bagel *(page 58)*

LUNCH .... Leftovers: Green Chili Baked Chicken + Lime Quinoa

DINNER .... Chimichurri Pork Tenderloin* *(page 108)*

+ Fresh Corn Salad Speckled with Cilantro* *(page 122)*

SNACK 1 .... 1 cup sliced cucumbers + 2 tablespoons tzatziki

SNACK 2 .... 3 tablespoons walnuts

FRIDAY

BREAKFAST .... Pomegranate Chia Pudding* *(page 52)*

LUNCH .... Leftovers: Chimichurri Pork Tenderloin

+ Fresh Corn Salad Speckled with Cilantro

DINNER .... Oven-Baked Chicken Shawarma* *(page 105)* + 1 whole-wheat pita bread

+ Marinated Cucumber and Tomato Salad *(page 146)*

SNACK 1 .... 1 hardboiled egg

SNACK 2 .... ½ avocado sprinkled with salt

SATURDAY

BRUNCH .... Spicy Chickpeas and Eggs over Arugula *(page 69)*

DINNER .... Leftovers: Oven-Baked Chicken Shawarma + 1 whole-wheat pita bread

+ Marinated Cucumber and Tomato Salad

SNACK 1 .... 1 apple + 1 tablespoon almond butter

SNACK 2 .... 1 cup leftover Pomegranate Chia Pudding

SUNDAY

BRUNCH .... Leftovers: Pomegranate Chia Pudding

topped with additional fruit, almond butter, and honey

DINNER .... Sheet Pan French Onion Chicken* *(page 106)*

+ Crispy Roasted Multicolored Baby Potatoes* *(page 127)*

SNACK 1 .... 1 cup carrots + 2 tablespoons tzatziki

SNACK 2 .... ½ whole-wheat bagel + ¼ avocado

WEEK TWO EXERCISE PLAN

You're ready to increase the intensity slightly. You will need a pair of 2-pound hand weights, or two household objects that are approximately 2 pounds and that you can easily hold in your hands, such as filled water bottles or candlesticks. If this seems too easy, you can move up to 5- or 10-pound weights. Complete one set of the core, upper body, lower body, and full body exercises, then take a break for water, and repeat for a total of two sets. Finish with some stretching of your choice, and remember to include a walk at some point in your day.

Core: *Dead Bug—Lie with your back on the floor and bend your knees so your feet are flat on the floor. Lift your bent legs until they are over your hips, and extend your arms halfway overhead, with your elbows bent. Now straighten one leg and the opposite arm, but don't let them touch the floor. Alternate with the other arm and leg. That's one repetition. Complete 10 for one set.*

Upper Body: *Shoulder Shrugs—Stand with your legs shoulder-width apart and a weight (whatever weight works for you) in each hand—or no weights, if you're not ready for them yet. Drop your arms to the sides of your body. Simply raise your shoulders 10 times for one set.*

Lower Body: *Squats—Stand with your feet shoulder-width apart. Lower your hips slowly into a squat, as if you were sitting on a chair, then stand back up. Complete 10 for one set.*

Full Body: *Weighted Jumping Jacks—With 2-pound weights in your hands—or no weights, if you're not ready for them yet—complete 10 jumping jacks for one set.*

Stretching: *After completing two sets of these four exercises, end your workout by stretching for 5 or more minutes.*

Cardio: *Walk—Take a briskly paced walk around the block or on a treadmill for 30 minutes.*

Week Three

As you've gotten into the swing of things, you probably have noticed how much easier meal preparation has become. You're saving time and money, plus you're improving your overall health and boosting your metabolism! This week, you'll be preparing a new seafood recipe and a vegetarian meal.

CANNED, BOTTLED, AND JARRED ITEMS

- Almond butter
- Black lentils, 1 (15-ounce) can
- Bruschetta spread, store-bought (½ cup)
- Marinara sauce (less than 260 mg of sodium per serving), 2 (12-ounce) jars
- Rice wine vinegar
- Sun-dried tomato pesto (¼ cup)

DAIRY AND EGGS

- Eggs (15)
- Parmesan cheese, grated (3 tablespoons)
- Yogurt, plain low-fat (2 cups)

MEAT, POULTRY, AND SEAFOOD

- Chicken breasts, boneless, skinless (8)
- Grass-fed beef sirloin (1 pound)
- Grass-fed flank steak, (1 pound)
- Salmon, 4 (6-ounce) fillets

PANTRY ITEMS

- Bread, whole-wheat (we like Ezekiel Bread or Dave's Killer Bread®) (6 slices)
- Brown rice, uncooked (1 cup)
- Cayenne pepper
- Chia seeds (1 tablespoon)
- Chickpea spaghetti, 1 (8-ounce) box
- Quinoa, uncooked (1½ cups)
- Hemp seeds, hulled (2 tablespoons)
- Sumac
- Thyme, dried

REFRIGERATED AND FROZEN ITEMS

- Chimichurri sauce (¼ cup)
- Hummus (1 package)
- Potatoes, frozen shredded (1 bag)

PRODUCE

- Arugula (1 cup)
- Asparagus (1 bunch)
- Avocados, medium (6)
- Bell peppers, green (2)
- Bell peppers, red (4)
- Carrots, whole (1 bag)
- Cauliflower (1 head)
- Cherry tomatoes (1 pint)
- Cucumbers, English (3)
- Garlic (8 cloves)
- Lemon (1)
- Limes (2)
- Onion, red, large (1)
- Onion, white (1)
- Onion, yellow, medium (1)
- Potatoes, baby, multicolored (8)
- Shallot (1)
- Spinach, fresh (3 cups)
- Strawberries (2 pints)
- Zucchini (1)

FRESH HERBS

- Rosemary, fresh
- Thyme, fresh

Meal substitutions:

» Grilled Salmon with Cilantro Yogurt Sauce (page 86) for Chimichurri Baked Salmon
» Frozen Breakfast Yogurt Pops (page 54) for Mediterranean Quinoa Breakfast Bowl

MONDAY

BREAKFAST	Sliced Strawberry and Nut Butter Sandwich (page 57)
LUNCH	Leftovers from Week Two: Sheet Pan French Onion Chicken + Crispy Roasted Multicolored Baby Potatoes
DINNER	Chimichurri Baked Salmon* (page 82) + ½ cup brown rice + Marinated Cucumber and Tomato Salad* (page 146)
SNACK 1	1 hardboiled egg
SNACK 2	1 cup sliced bell pepper

TUESDAY

BREAKFAST	Loaded Hash Brown Vegetable Frittata Cups (page 70)
LUNCH	Leftovers: Chimichurri Baked Salmon + ½ cup brown rice + Marinated Cucumber and Tomato Salad
DINNER	Herb-Baked Steak Bites* (page 111) + Parmesan Roasted Carrots* (page 119)
SNACK 1	½ avocado sprinkled with sea salt
SNACK 2	1 cup strawberries

WEDNESDAY

BREAKFAST	Sliced Strawberry and Nut Butter Sandwich (page 57)
LUNCH	Leftovers: Herb-Baked Steak Bites + Parmesan Roasted Carrots
DINNER	Chili Lime Chicken* (page 98) + Grilled Avocado Stuffed with Lentil Salad* (page 133)
SNACK 1	1 cup sliced bell pepper
SNACK 2	1 cup cucumbers + 2 tablespoons hummus

THURSDAY

BREAKFAST .... Loaded Hash Brown Vegetable Frittata Cups *(page 70)*
LUNCH .... Leftovers: Chili Lime Chicken
+ Grilled Avocado Stuffed with Lentil Salad
DINNER .... Sheet Pan Steak Fajitas* *(page 113)* + ½ cup brown rice
SNACK 1 .... 1 cup strawberries
SNACK 2 .... 1 cup cauliflower dipped in 1 tablespoon chimichurri sauce

FRIDAY

BREAKFAST .... Sliced Strawberry and Nut Butter Sandwich *(page 57)*
LUNCH .... Leftovers: Sheet Pan Steak Fajitas + ½ cup brown rice
DINNER .... Fragrant Sumac Chicken * *(page 100)* + ½ cup quinoa
+ 1 cup steamed asparagus
SNACK 1 .... 1 cup cucumbers + 2 tablespoons hummus
SNACK 2 .... ½ avocado sprinkled with sea salt

SATURDAY

BRUNCH .... Mediterranean Quinoa Breakfast Bowl *(page 60)*
DINNER .... Leftovers: Fragrant Sumac Chicken
+ ½ cup quinoa + 1 cup steamed asparagus
SNACK 1 .... 1 slice whole-wheat toast + 1 tablespoon almond butter
SNACK 2 .... 1 cup carrots + ¼ cup hummus

SUNDAY

BRUNCH .... Eat the Rainbow Veggie Scramble *(page 64)*
DINNER .... Protein-Packed Chickpea Spaghetti* *(page 131)*
SNACK 1 .... 1 cup plain low-fat yogurt topped with 1 tablespoon almond butter
SNACK 2 .... 1 slice whole-wheat toast + ¼ avocado

Once again, you will be increasing the difficulty of the exercises ever so slightly. You will need a pair of 2-pound hand weights, or two household objects that are approximately 2 pounds and that you can easily hold in your hands. If this seems too easy, you can move up to 5- or 10-pound weights. Complete one set of the core, upper body, lower body, and full body exercises, then take a break for water, and repeat for a total of two sets. Finish with some stretching of your choice, and remember to include a walk at some point in your day.

Core: *Boat—Sit on the ground with your knees bent and your feet on the floor. Hug under your thighs, right above the knees. Lean back, and your feet will come off the floor. Your shins should now be parallel to the floor, and your upper body should be at about a 45-degree angle to the floor. In this position, with your palms facing up, extend your arms in front of you at shoulder height. Hold for 30 seconds.*

Upper Body: *Shoulder Press—With a 2-pound weight in each hand (or whatever weight works for you), hold your arms at shoulder height and bend your elbows so your arms are at right angles and your hands are level with your head. Lift the weights up and slowly lower them down to the starting position. That's one repetition. Complete 5 for one set.*

Lower Body: *Side Leg Raises—Stand with your legs together. Keeping one leg straight, extend the other leg to your side. Alternate left and right for a total of 30 raises. That's one set.*

Full Body: *Mountain Climbers—With both hands and feet flat on the ground (kind of like the way a bear walks on all fours), rise up to the tips of your toes. In this position, quickly pull your right leg to your right elbow, then quickly do the same with your left. That's one repetition. Complete 10 for one set.*

Stretching: *Now that you have completed three weeks of exercise, stretching is ever so important. After completing two sets of these four exercises, end your workout by stretching effectively for 5 or more minutes.*

Cardio: *Walk or Light Jog—Since you've been building up your stamina and cardiovascular health, feel free to turn this 30-minute walk into a light jog, or a combination of the two.*

Week Four

Wow! You're already at week four and we bet you're feeling incredible. We hope you've become more in tune with your fullness and hunger cues, and learned that eating every few hours helps mitigate food cravings. You've probably also realized that although these recipes are super healthy, they're extremely delicious, too. We've saved some of our favorite recipes for last, including our Matcha Meyer Lemon Ricotta Crêpes and Miso-Glazed Chicken.

SHOPPING LIST

CANNED, BOTTLED, AND JARRED ITEMS

- Agave nectar, pure (1 teaspoon)
- Cooking sherry *also*, Sesame oil
- Tomatoes, diced, low-sodium, 1 (14.5-ounce) can

DAIRY AND EGGS

- Eggs (18)
- Greek yogurt, plain 2 percent, 1 (32-ounce) container
- Milk, 1 percent (1 cup)
- Ricotta cheese, low-fat (1½ cups)

MEAT, POULTRY, AND FISH

- Chicken breasts, boneless, skinless (8)
- Chicken tenders (1 pound)
- Grass-fed beef, lean ground (1 pound)
- Grass-fed flank steak (1 pound)
- Pink salmon, 1 (14.75-ounce) can
- Shrimp, fresh (1 pound)

PANTRY ITEMS

- Brown rice, uncooked (1 cup)
- Cashews, raw, unsalted (1 cup)
- Coriander, ground
- Curry powder (¼ cup)
- English muffins, whole-wheat (1 package)
- Farro, uncooked (1 cup)
- Hemp seeds, hulled (1 cup)
- Matcha powder, unsweetened (1 teaspoon)
- Pastry flour, whole-wheat (1 cup)
- Quinoa, uncooked (½ cup)

- Rolled oats,
  uncooked
  (2 cups)
- Sesame seeds
  (4 teaspoons)
- Tortillas,
  whole-wheat
  or gluten-free
  (we like La
  Tortilla Factory),
  4 (100-calorie)

REFRIGERATED AND FROZEN ITEMS

- Chimichurri sauce
  (2 tablespoons)
- Miso paste, white
  (½ cup)

PRODUCE

- Arugula (3 cups)
- Asparagus spears
  (1 pound)
- Avocados,
  medium (3)
- Bananas, large (5)
- Bok choy
  (1 pound)
- Carrots, large (2)
- English cucumber,
  large (1)
- Fennel bulbs (2)
- Garlic, 2 heads
- Ginger, 2 (3-inch)
  pieces
- Lemons (2)
- Lemon, Meyer (1)
- Onion, red (1)
- Onion, Vidalia,
  medium (or yellow
  onion) (1)
- Onions, white,
  medium (3)
- Spinach, 2
  (1-pound) bags
- Sweet potatoes,
  medium (9)
- Swiss chard,
  1 bunch
- Tomato (1)

FRESH HERBS

- Rosemary, fresh

WEEK FOUR MEAL PLAN

Meal substitutions:

» Italian-Style Salmon in Foil Packs for Garlic Fennel Shrimp
» Sumac and Cayenne Spiced Scallops for Spiced Beef Kebabs

MONDAY

BREAKFAST	Avocado Spinach Breakfast Burrito *(page 67)*
LUNCH	Leftovers from Week Three: Protein-Packed Chickpea Spaghetti
DINNER	Rosemary Lemon Chicken* *(page 96)*
	+ Roasted Asparagus* *(page 118)*
SNACK 1	3 tablespoons unsalted cashews
SNACK 2	1 banana

TUESDAY

BREAKFAST	Easy Banana Oat Pancakes *(page 62)*
LUNCH	Leftovers: Rosemary Lemon Chicken + Roasted Asparagus
DINNER	Garlic Fennel Shrimp* *(page 90)*
	+ Mediterranean Farro Salad* *(page 137)*
SNACK 1	1 cup plain low-fat Greek yogurt sprinkled with cinnamon
SNACK 2	1 hardboiled egg

WEDNESDAY

BREAKFAST	Avocado Spinach Breakfast Burrito *(page 67)*
LUNCH	Leftovers: Garlic Fennel Shrimp + Mediterranean Farro Salad
DINNER	Mediterranean Spiced Beef Meatballs* *(page 114)*
	+ Sweet Potatoes Stuffed with Swiss Chard* *(page 129)*
SNACK 1	1 cup sliced carrots
SNACK 2	½ cup cooked oatmeal + 1 tablespoon hulled hemp seeds

THURSDAY

BREAKFAST .... Easy Banana Oat Pancakes *(page 62)*

LUNCH .... Leftovers: Mediterranean Spiced Beef Meatballs
+ Sweet Potatoes Stuffed with Swiss Chard

DINNER .... Cashew Chicken Curry in a Hurry* *(page 104)*
+ Roasted Sesame Bok Choy* *(page 120)* + ½ cup brown rice

SNACK 1 .... 1 banana

SNACK 2 .... ½ cup plain low-fat Greek yogurt + 1 tablespoon hulled hemp seeds

FRIDAY

BREAKFAST .... Avocado Spinach Breakfast Burrito *(page 67)*

LUNCH .... Leftovers: Cashew Chicken Curry in a Hurry
+ Roasted Sesame Bok Choy + ½ cup brown rice

DINNER .... Spiced Beef Kebabs* *(page 115)*
+ Roasted Sesame Sweet Potatoes * *(page 128)*

SNACK 1 .... ½ cup low-fat ricotta cheese + 1 teaspoon cinnamon

SNACK 2 .... 1 cup sliced carrots

SATURDAY

BRUNCH .... Matcha Meyer Lemon Ricotta Crêpes *(page 63)*

DINNER .... Leftovers: Spiced Beef Kebabs + Roasted Sesame Sweet Potatoes

SNACK 1 .... 1 cup plain low-fat Greek yogurt sprinkled with cinnamon

SNACK 2 .... ½ cup cooked oatmeal + 2 tablespoons hulled hemp seeds

SUNDAY

BRUNCH .... Deconstructed Salmon Eggs Benedict *(page 71)*

DINNER .... Miso-Glazed Chicken *(page 103)* + ½ cup quinoa + steamed spinach

SNACK 1 .... ½ whole-wheat English muffin + ¼ avocado

SNACK 2 .... 3 tablespoons unsalted cashews + 1 banana

Consider this a recovery week! Repeat the same exercises you did in week one. We want to make sure your body is able to recover and does not become too strained.

FOUR-WEEK EXERCISE PLAN

The following chart summarizes your exercises for each week. Each week's routine consists of four days of workouts, two days of rest, and one day of an exercise of choice. You may wish to change which days you work out and which days you rest.

	WEEK 1	WEEK 2	WEEK 3	WEEK 4
	Two sets of each exercise **30 minutes walking (even on rest days)**	**Two sets of each exercise** **30 minutes walking (even on rest days)**	**Two sets of each exercise** **30 minutes walking (even on rest days)**	**Two sets of each exercise** **30 minutes walking (even on rest days)**
M	30 seconds plank 10 arm scissors 10 forward lunges 3 burpees	10 dead bugs 10 shoulder shrugs 10 squats 10 weighted jumping jacks	30 seconds boat 5 shoulder presses 30 side leg raises 10 mountain climbers	30 seconds plank 10 arm scissors 10 forward lunges 3 burpees
T	30 seconds plank 10 arm scissors 10 forward lunges 3 burpees	10 dead bugs 10 shoulder shrugs 10 squats 10 weighted jumping jacks	30 seconds boat 5 shoulder presses 30 side leg raises 10 mountain climbers	30 seconds plank 10 arm scissors 10 forward lunges 3 burpees
W	REST	REST	REST	REST
T	30 seconds plank 10 arm scissors 10 forward lunges 3 burpees	10 dead bugs 10 shoulder shrugs 10 squats 10 weighted jumping jacks	30 seconds boat 5 shoulder presses 30 side leg raises 10 mountain climbers	30 seconds plank 10 arm scissors 10 forward lunges 3 burpees
F	30 seconds plank 10 arm scissors 10 forward lunges 3 burpees	10 dead bugs 10 shoulder shrugs 10 squats 10 weighted jumping jacks	30 seconds plank 10 arm scissors 10 forward lunges 3 burpees	30 seconds plank 10 arm scissors 10 forward lunges 3 burpees
S	REST	REST	REST	REST
S	Exercise of choice: tennis, group class, swimming, etc.	Exercise of choice	Exercise of choice	Exercise of choice

After Four Weeks

Congratulations! You have officially completed our four-week fast metabolism diet plan! We bet you are feeling healthy, accomplished, and energized. Now it's time for us to sit down and discuss the plan moving forward.

You've probably heard many times in your life that lifestyle change is key for long-term success. Well, it's totally true! The reason strict diets don't work long-term is that they aren't personalized to fit your unique lifestyle. Since you will be making your own meal plans moving forward, you will know exactly what does and doesn't work for you.

When developing your meal plans, keep in mind that lifestyle change allows for some wiggle room—meaning you don't have to be perfect. We like our clients to follow the 80/20 rule: If you eat well 80 percent or more of the time and indulge 20 percent or less of the time, you're on the right track. In addition, remember that it's normal to fall off the wagon sometimes, especially when you're on vacation or during a special celebration. If this happens (and know that it will), we encourage you to get back on track as soon as you can. The trick is to not let a four-day vacation turn into a four-week binge.

Also, remember that feeling guilty after indulging is *not* okay and is not helpful! Having treat foods like cake, pizza, and wine is good for the soul, especially when you are enjoying these with friends and family. We also find that people who feel excessive guilt tend to be more likely to binge eat.

While you are creating your shopping lists and meal plans, keep in mind how amazing you have been feeling while on this four-week plan. Notice that you did not consume any alcohol, caffeine, refined or artificial sugars, or other processed foods like chips, candy, and soda. You may choose to continue avoiding these foods. If you decide to reintroduce, say, candy, why not shop for a healthier version? For example, instead of buying a generic peanut butter cup, why not get a dark chocolate almond butter cup? You might enjoy it even more. This is your time to think outside the box, break old habits, and try new things. Instead of going back to drinking soda, how about sparkling water with a splash of lime? Instead of drinking a cup of coffee in the morning, why not try a decaf cup of herbal tea? The possibilities are endless.

As you may know, your taste buds do change over time. As you begin to eat healthier, you will find that you prefer certain flavors over others. Since we've cut artificial sweeteners like sucralose and xylitol out of your diet, you may become more aware of their chemical-like flavor the next time you eat a sugar-free protein bar.

Long-term lifestyle changes must include variety. Continue to cook your favorite recipes from this book but also consider modifying your old go-to recipes. For instance, if a recipe calls for white flour, substitute almond flour or whole-wheat flour. If you'd like to continue avoiding soy, substitute coconut aminos for soy sauce.

Last but not least, our four-week reset addressed lifestyle factors such as sleep, water intake, and exercise. As you've probably experienced, when you are getting enough sleep, your sugar cravings go down tremendously. We want you to be the most successful you can be. Therefore, we highly encourage you to continue prioritizing sleep.

In terms of water, being dehydrated significantly lowers energy levels and makes it more difficult for your body to properly digest and absorb the nutrients from your food. Do the best you can to continue drinking plenty of water, decaf teas, sparkling water, and other hydrating beverages. Exercise ties everything together and improves your sleep, stress levels, and mood. Find the exercises you love and stick with them!

Planning Your Week

You will be designing your own meal plans based on your taste buds and lifestyle. The key to long-term success is finding something that you personally can stick with for good. That means if you love desserts like we do, be sure to include dessert items on your shopping list each week. If you know you get really hungry in the afternoon, be sure to include two or three afternoon snacks in your plan. If you work out harder on the weekends, make sure to plan for a larger lunch and dinner to help you recover and fill your belly. Here are some more suggestions for planning your week.

FOLLOW THE GOLDEN RULE

When writing your own weekly meal plan, always remember to include carbohydrates, proteins, and fats in every meal. People often undervalue the importance of complex carbohydrates and fats when trying to lose weight and boost metabolism. But the body needs both of these macronutrients just as much as it needs protein to function at its best. With every meal, try to shoot for a plate that looks like this: chicken breast, sweet potato, and greens topped with olive oil.

STAY ORGANIZED!

Bring a grocery list to the store with you to avoid purchasing impulse items (such as tempting desserts or snacks). In addition, this will expedite your shopping trip, saving you time. We also recommend using the blank meal plan on page 160 and writing down all your meals for the week. Place this on your refrigerator to use as a menu.

WHAT'S IN MY REFRIGERATOR?

When deciding what meals to prepare for the week, look through your refrigerator and pantry to see what you already have. Use these foods to come up with recipes for your meal plan. For instance, if you have frozen broccoli and rice, why not make a teriyaki chicken and rice bowl with veggies for dinner that week? Checking through your refrigerator and pantry first will help cut down on costs and minimize food waste.

VEGGIES FOR BREAKFAST

Try to incorporate vegetables into every meal. They are packed with essential vitamins, minerals, and fiber, and play a huge role in detoxifying the body and resetting your metabolism. We understand, however, that it can be difficult to include vegetables with particular meals, such as breakfast. Most of our breakfast recipes incorporate vegetables, so we recommend using these as a good first start. Then you can come up with your own creative ways to incorporate veggies with breakfast.

GANG UP ON THE MEAL PREP

Pick two days per week to prepare all your meals, and mark them down in your calendar. Check your schedule and make a note of busy days when you can plan to eat leftovers. We find that people who set time aside to cook are the most successful. It will also make life a lot easier when you are in a rush and need to grab and go. Having food already prepared also minimizes your craving to dine out or order takeout.

FROZEN IS JUST AS GOOD

The time needed to prepare fresh fruits and vegetables can add up, so we recommend buying frozen organic produce when you can. Frozen fruits and veggies contain the same nutritional value as their fresh counterparts, and in some cases are even more nutritious. This is because they are typically picked when they are at their ripest, meaning that the highest amount of nutrients and vitamins are available. Another bonus about buying frozen fruits and veggies is that they don't go bad, saving you money.

VARIETY IS THE BEST SPICE

Make a weekly meal plan that includes variety. It's common to prepare meals for several days using a limited set of ingredients: Think about those chicken, brown rice, and broccoli folks you know. But the lack of variety might result in excluding other essential nutrients. Additionally, it is very easy to grow bored with repetitive meals. The last thing we want is for you to not enjoy your food and lose motivation.

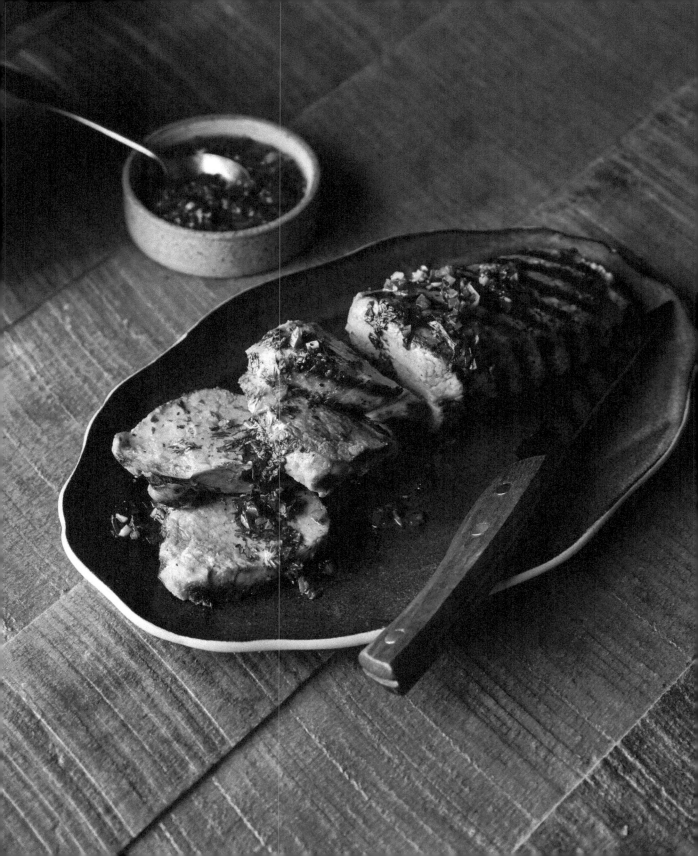

PART TWO

FAST METABOLISM RECIPES

As promised, all our recipes incorporate metabolism-boosting ingredients to make the magic happen. Unlike fad diets or low-calorie meal plans that restrict food and nutrients your body needs, our recipes contain powerful vitamins, minerals, and antioxidants that will help you feel more vibrant and lighter on your feet. Many of our recipes include additional details about how the ingredients speed up your metabolic rate. And remember, not only are the recipes healthy, they truly taste delicious. Trust us—we've tried them all.

CHIMICHURRI PORK TENDERLOIN, PAGE 108

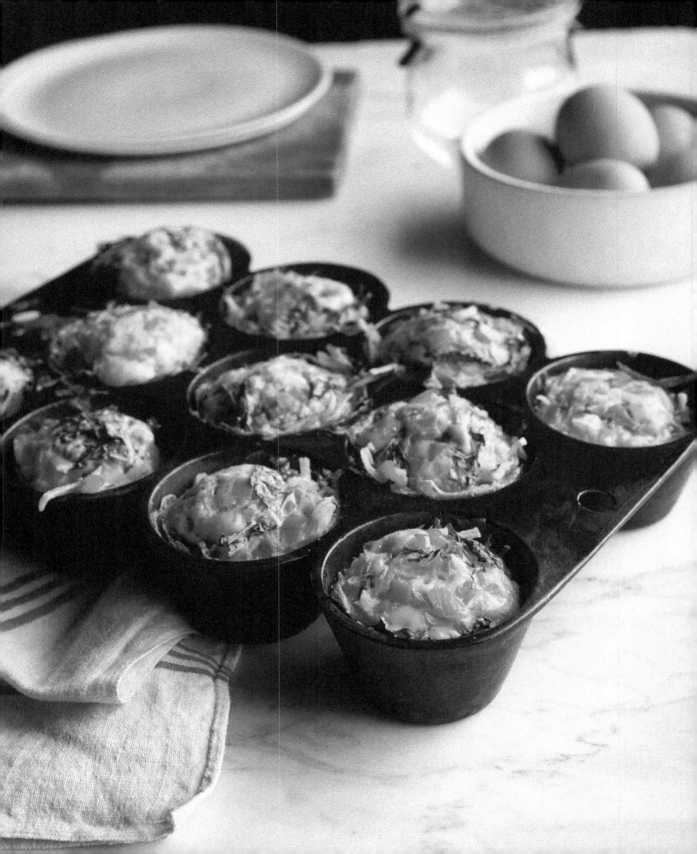

CHAPTER 3

Breakfast and Brunch

Pomegranate Chia Pudding

SERVES 2 / PREP TIME: 10 MINUTES, PLUS 2 HOURS TO CHILL

Chia seeds contain lots of omega-3 fatty acids, protein, fiber, and minerals; coconut milk has a lot of healthy fats; and pomegranate juice is antioxidant-rich. Together, they make this a great nutrient-dense snack or meal for any time of the day. You can buy hulled hemp seeds, also called hemp hearts, at most grocery stores or online. They have a slightly nutty taste and are a great, sustainable source of plant-based protein. Plus, they are high in omega-3 and omega-6 fats, which are great for brain and heart health.

1 cup unsweetened coconut milk

1 cup pomegranate juice

4 tablespoons chia seeds

2 tablespoons hulled hemp seeds

1. Pour ½ cup of unsweetened coconut milk and ½ cup of pomegranate juice in each of two medium plastic containers or glass jars.

2. Add 2 tablespoons of chia seeds and 1 tablespoon of hemp seeds to each container and stir thoroughly until well combined.

3. Cover and store in the refrigerator for 2 hours or overnight.

STORAGE TIP: For a quick breakfast, double the recipe and store in the refrigerator for up to four days. For variety, top the pudding with unsweetened coconut flakes or homemade granola.

Per Serving: Calories: 242; Fat: 14g; Saturated Fat: 3g; Sodium: 28mg; Cholesterol: 0mg; Carbs: 26g; Fiber: 14g; Sugar: 20g; Protein: 12g

Papaya Greek Yogurt Bowl

SERVES 2 / PREP TIME: 5 MINUTES / COOK TIME: 3 MINUTES

Papaya contains a powerful digestive enzyme called papain. This delicious recipe can help improve digestion and detoxify the body of harmful toxins that could be slowing down your metabolic rate. You can find chia seeds at most grocery stores or online. They have a mild flavor and look very similar to poppy seeds. Chia seeds are high in fiber, aiding in gut health.

4 tablespoons unsalted sliced almonds

2 cups plain low-fat Greek yogurt

1 teaspoon pure vanilla extract

2 teaspoons fresh lemon juice

1 teaspoon honey

1 small papaya, cut in half and seeded

2 teaspoons chia seeds

1. Toast the almonds by heating them in a dry skillet over medium-high heat. Watch the almonds closely and stir occasionally, because they will brown in as little as 2 to 3 minutes.

2. In a medium bowl, mix together the Greek yogurt, vanilla, lemon juice, and honey.

3. Spoon the yogurt mixture into each papaya half and top both with 2 tablespoons of toasted almonds and 1 teaspoon of chia seeds.

VARIATION: You can substitute small honeydew melon or cantaloupe halves for the papaya.

Per Serving: Calories: 316; Fat: 10g; Saturated Fat: 1g; Sodium: 124mg; Cholesterol: 4mg; Carbs: 28g; Fiber: 6g; Sugar: 19g; Protein: 28g

Frozen Breakfast Yogurt Pops

MAKES 10 POPS (2 OR 3 PER SERVING) / PREP TIME: 12 MINUTES, PLUS 4 HOURS TO FREEZE

Berries are packed with antioxidants and help naturally sweeten this protein-packed breakfast. Granola gives a satisfying crunch to these delectable pops. The paper cups make for a more convenient on-the-go breakfast with no cleanup. If you want to keep these pops in the freezer for up to four days, freeze the yogurt mixture in ice-pop molds.

½ cup unsweetened coconut milk

1½ cups low-fat plain Greek yogurt

2 teaspoons honey

1½ cups frozen mixed berries

10 medium paper cups

1 cup matcha granola (from Baked Peaches Topped with Matcha Granola, page 157)

1. In a medium bowl, mix the coconut milk, yogurt, honey, and berries until the berries begin to break down and the yogurt mixture has slightly changed color from the berries, 1 to 2 minutes.

2. To assemble, line up the paper cups on a baking sheet. Fill the bottom of each paper cup with a dollop of the yogurt mixture. Layer with granola and top with remaining yogurt, leaving ½ inch of space at the top of the cup.

3. Cover the paper cups with plastic wrap and freeze until firm, about 4 hours. Gently peel the paper cup away from the pop to enjoy.

INGREDIENT TIP: You can substitute store-bought granola for homemade, but be careful: Commercial granolas are often loaded with sugar. Pick one with fewer than 6 grams of sugar per serving.

Per Serving: Calories: 168; Fat: 14g; Saturated Fat: 6g; Sodium: 46mg; Cholesterol: 2mg; Carbs: 29g; Fiber: 5g; Sugar: 15g; Protein: 13g

Carrot Cake Overnight Oats with Flax and Walnuts

SERVES 2 / PREP TIME: 15 MINUTES, PLUS OVERNIGHT TO CHILL

These overnight oats taste amazingly close to the cooked kind, plus they help you incorporate vegetables into your morning meal. Protein comes from the cow's milk, while walnuts and flaxseeds provide omega-3 fatty acids. As a time-saver, you can double the recipe and store in glass containers in the refrigerator for up to four days for a grab-and-go breakfast option.

1 cup uncooked whole-grain rolled oats

1 cup 1-percent milk

2 large carrots, peeled and finely shredded

½ teaspoon cinnamon

2 tablespoons ground flaxseeds

½ cup coarsely chopped walnuts

1. Place ½ cup of oats in each of two medium glass or plastic containers.
2. Into each container, pour ½ cup of milk and add 1 finely shredded carrot, ¼ teaspoon of cinnamon, and 1 tablespoon of ground flaxseeds. Stir well. Top each mixture with ¼ cup of walnuts.
3. Cover with the lid and refrigerate overnight.

VARIATION: If you are lactose intolerant, sensitive to dairy, or vegan, swap any non-dairy milk substitute for the cow's milk.

Per Serving: Calories: 456; Fat: 24g; Saturated Fat: 4g; Sodium: 107mg; Cholesterol: 6mg; Carbs: 46g; Fiber: 10g; Sugar: 11g; Protein: 15g

Apple Cinnamon Oatmeal

SERVES 2 / PREP TIME: 10 MINUTES / COOK TIME: 15 MINUTES

Oats are a great source of fiber and provide a steady release of energy throughout the morning. The apple's natural sugars and the warm, sweet flavor of the cinnamon allow you to enjoy a tasty breakfast without using added sweeteners. Add a pinch of salt to the oatmeal to bring out the sweetness of the apples even more.

Avocado oil spray

1 apple, unpeeled, washed, cored, and finely chopped

1 teaspoon cinnamon

1¾ cups water

1 cup uncooked whole-grain rolled oats

2 tablespoons hulled hemp seeds

½ cup coarsely chopped walnuts

1. Coat a medium saucepan with avocado oil and heat over medium heat.

2. Add the apple and cinnamon and cook 4 to 5 minutes, stirring, until the apples begin to break down. Add the water and bring to a boil.

3. Stir in the oats and cook for about 5 minutes over medium heat, stirring occasionally.

4. Stir again before serving, and top each serving with 1 tablespoon of hemp seeds and ¼ cup of walnuts.

STORAGE TIP: For a quick and convenient breakfast, double the recipe and store in glass containers in the refrigerator for up to three days.

Per Serving: Calories: 391; Fat: 17g; Saturated Fat: 2g; Sodium: 3mg; Cholesterol: 0mg; Carbs: 48g; Fiber: 10g; Sugar: 12g; Protein: 12g

Sliced Strawberry and Nut Butter Sandwich

SERVES 2 / PREP TIME: 5 MINUTES

This spin on a classic PB&J replaces store-bought jelly with fresh strawberries. Hemp and chia seeds provide protein and healthy fatty acids to leave you feeling much fuller and more satisfied than the original. Make sure you choose a whole-grain bread; our favorites include Ezekiel Bread and Dave's Killer Bread®. And pick an almond butter that contains only almonds and/or salt—read the labels carefully.

4 slices whole-wheat bread

4 tablespoons natural almond butter

2 tablespoons hulled hemp seeds

1 tablespoon chia seeds

5 large strawberries, sliced

1. Toast the bread the way you like it. Spread 1 tablespoon of almond butter on each slice of toast.

2. Sprinkle 2 of the slices of bread with 1 tablespoon of hemp seeds, ½ tablespoon of chia seeds, and the sliced strawberries. Top with the other 2 slices of bread.

3. Serve immediately or wrap in foil and store in the refrigerator for up to two days.

VARIATION: You can switch in any fruit you have on hand. A great option would be sliced apples or mashed raspberries.

Per Serving: Calories: 478; Fat: 28g; Saturated Fat: 3g; Sodium: 330mg; Cholesterol: 0mg; Carbs: 35g; Fiber: 13g; Sugar: 7g; Protein: 22g

Avocado and Lox Bagel

SERVES 2 / PREP TIME: 6 MINUTES

Salmon is a great source of iron, zinc, niacin, vitamin B_6, vitamin B_{12}, and other nutrients you need for a healthy metabolism, making it one of the healthiest fish you can eat. Choose foods and products that are naturally colored and try to avoid purchasing foods that contain dyes, as they are thought to be carcinogenic. Good-quality lox won't contain additives and will specify whether it was farmed or wild-caught. Choose Alaskan wild-caught salmon, which tends to be lower in mercury and richer in omega-3 fatty acids.

1 medium ripe avocado

1 teaspoon fresh lemon juice

Salt

Freshly ground black pepper

2 whole-wheat everything bagels (we like Ezekiel Bread)

6 ounces lox

2 thin slices red onion

4 thin slices tomato

1 teaspoon capers, rinsed

1. In small bowl, mash the avocado with the lemon juice and season with a pinch of salt and pepper.

2. Split the bagels in half and toast. Once toasted, top each half with equal amounts of the avocado mixture and layer with lox, onion, tomato, and capers.

3. Serve sandwich-style or open-faced. Serve immediately or store for up to a few hours in the refrigerator.

VARIATION: Use lemon pepper or garlic salt instead of salt and pepper. This dish would also be great with sliced cucumber and fresh spinach.

Per Serving: Calories: 365; Fat: 18g; Saturated Fat: 3g; Sodium: 2010mg; Cholesterol: 20mg; Carbs: 31g; Fiber: 13g; Sugar: 4g; Protein: 23g

Balanced Breakfast Sandwich

SERVES 2 / PREP TIME: 5 MINUTES / COOK TIME: 2 MINUTES

We think you will love this Balanced Breakfast Sandwich. The whole-wheat muffins and arugula provide stomach-filling fiber to keep your blood sugar stable. And, as a bonus, microwaving the eggs and bacon makes for amazingly fast prep in the morning. Nitrates in bacon are used in the curing process to preserve the meat and prevent bacteria from growing. Some research, however, has found that nitrates are carcinogenic.

2 whole-wheat English muffins

2 eggs

Salt

Freshly ground black pepper

4 slices nitrate-free Canadian bacon

1 cup fresh spinach

1. Split and toast the English muffins.
2. Crack the eggs into two small glass containers and season with salt and pepper. Poke the yolks with a fork. Microwave on high for 1 minute, or until firm. Slide the eggs onto two English muffin halves.
3. Place the Canadian bacon on a microwaveable plate and microwave on high for 1 minute, or until heated. Place on top of the eggs.
4. Top each sandwich with ½ cup of fresh spinach and other English muffin half. Serve immediately.

STORAGE TIP: Wrap an English muffin sandwich in a paper towel and then in foil. Place in a zip-top bag and store in the freezer for up to 1 month. To reheat, remove the foil and microwave the frozen sandwich in the paper towel for 2 to 3 minutes, or until hot.

Per Serving: Calories: 316; Fat: 8g; Saturated Fat: 3g; Sodium: 1213mg; Cholesterol: 214mg; Carbs: 28g; Fiber: 2g; Sugar: 4g; Protein: 31g

Mediterranean Quinoa Breakfast Bowl

SERVES 2 / PREP TIME: 6 MINUTES / COOK TIME: 5 MINUTES

Mixing creamy and savory yields a unique yet delicious combination of flavors. Protein from the yogurt and eggs, fat from the pesto, carbohydrates from the quinoa, and fiber from the leafy greens make for a well-rounded meal that will fuel you for hours.

1 teaspoon avocado oil

2 eggs

1 cup plain low-fat Greek yogurt

¼ cup store-bought sun-dried tomato pesto

Salt

Freshly ground black pepper

1 cup cooked quinoa

1 cup fresh spinach

1. Heat the oil in a medium skillet over medium-high heat. When the oil is hot, add the eggs and cook as you like them.

2. In a medium bowl, mix together the Greek yogurt, pesto, and a pinch of salt and pepper. Divide between two bowls.

3. Spoon the cooked quinoa over the yogurt. Top each with ½ cup of spinach and one egg.

VARIATION: Try basil or cilantro pesto to change the flavor profile of the yogurt. Top with additional seasonings, such as fresh herbs, sesame seeds, red pepper flakes, or lemon zest.

Per Serving: Calories: 280; Fat: 10g; Saturated Fat: 2g; Sodium: 286mg; Cholesterol: 167mg; Carbs: 27g; Fiber: 3g; Sugar: 6g; Protein: 22g

Hearty Farro, Yogurt, and Egg Bowl

SERVES 2 / PREP TIME: 6 MINUTES / COOK TIME: 5 MINUTES

This bowl hits all the macronutrient components of a balanced diet and will fuel you for any morning task. Farro is a hearty grain that has a slightly nutty flavor. It looks a lot like barley and is cooked similarly to rice. Farro provides a satisfying amount of complex carbohydrates that will keep you full throughout your morning. To add variety, sprinkle with no-salt-added everything bagel seasoning or chopped fresh herbs such as cilantro, basil, or dill.

1 teaspoon avocado oil

2 eggs

1 cup plain low-fat Greek yogurt

Zest and juice of 1 lemon

Salt

Freshly ground black pepper

1 cup cooked farro

1 large avocado, sliced

1 cup fresh arugula

Red pepper flakes

1. Heat the oil in a medium skillet over medium-high heat. When the oil is hot, add the eggs and cook as you like them.

2. In a medium bowl, mix together the Greek yogurt and half the lemon zest, and season with salt and pepper.

3. Divide the yogurt between two bowls or glass storage containers. Top each with ½ cup of cooked farro, one egg, and half of the avocado.

4. Top each bowl with ½ cup of arugula, half the lemon zest, the lemon juice, and a pinch of red pepper flakes.

VARIATION: To save time, use some leftover Lime Quinoa (page 134) instead of farro.

Per Serving: Calories: 412; Fat: 19g; Saturated Fat: 4g; Sodium: 136mg; Cholesterol: 166mg; Carbs: 39g; Fiber: 8g; Sugar: 6g; Protein: 24g

Easy Banana Oat Pancakes

SERVES 2 / PREP TIME: 5 MINUTES / COOK TIME: 10 MINUTES

These pancakes are fast, nutritious, and won't leave you reaching for the syrup. Bananas and uncooked oats are a great source of resistance fiber (also known as indigestible fiber), which has been shown to promote weight loss and weight maintenance. For additional protein, top these pancakes with a dollop of Greek yogurt.

2 large ripe bananas

2 eggs

1 teaspoon pure vanilla extract

½ cup uncooked rolled oats

2 tablespoons hulled hemp seeds

1 teaspoon cinnamon, plus a pinch more

1 teaspoon coconut oil

1. Mash the bananas in a large bowl with a fork or a potato masher until smooth. Stir in the eggs and vanilla extract. Add the oats, hemp seeds, and cinnamon, and mix until well combined.

2. Heat the coconut oil in a medium pan over medium heat. Wait for the pan to get hot and then pour in ½ cup of the pancake batter.

3. Cook for 2 to 3 minutes, until you see bubbles forming on top of the batter. Flip and cook until the other side is golden brown, 1 to 2 minutes. Repeat until you have used up all the pancake batter.

4. Sprinkle the pancakes with a pinch of cinnamon and serve immediately.

PREPARATION TIP: To get the right consistency and sweetness, it is key to use ripe bananas that are very yellow with lots of brown spots on the peel.

Per Serving: Calories: 377; Fat: 14g; Saturated Fat: 5g; Sodium: 64mg; Cholesterol: 163mg; Carbs: 49g; Fiber: 8g; Sugar: 18g; Protein: 15g

Matcha Meyer Lemon Ricotta Crêpes

SERVES 3 (2 CRÊPES PER SERVING) / PREP TIME: 8 MINUTES / COOK TIME: 12 MINUTES

This matcha crêpe will energize you naturally, so you don't need that cup of coffee. Matcha is made from green tea leaves that have been ground into a powder. It may offer a variety of health benefits, including preventing heart disease and aiding in weight loss, according to several studies. Try dusting the finished crêpes with extra matcha powder and serve with a slice of lemon.

For the filling

1 cup low-fat ricotta cheese

Juice of 1 medium Meyer lemon

1 teaspoon agave nectar

1 teaspoon pure vanilla extract

For the crêpes

1 cup whole-wheat pastry flour

3 eggs

1 cup 1-percent milk

1 teaspoon agave nectar

1 teaspoon pure vanilla extract

1 teaspoon unsweetened matcha powder

¼ teaspoon salt

Avocado oil spray

To make the filling

1. In a medium bowl, mix ricotta cheese, Meyer lemon juice, agave nectar, and vanilla extract together until smooth.
2. Set aside while you make the crêpes.

To make the crêpes

1. Place pastry flour, eggs, milk, agave nectar, vanilla extract, matcha powder, and salt in a large bowl and mix well.
2. Spray a medium sauté pan or skillet with avocado oil for 1 second and heat over medium heat.
3. Pour ¼ cup of the batter into the pan. Very quickly swirl the batter around to cover the pan in one thin layer. After 1 minute, when the batter starts to set and slightly curl up from the edge of the pan, carefully flip it over without tearing the crêpe. Cook for 1 more minute on the other side until it is golden brown, and transfer to plate. Repeat until there is no batter remaining.
4. Fill each crêpe with 2 tablespoons of the filling mixture and roll up. Serve immediately.

VARIATION: Use regular lemons if Meyer lemons are not available or in season.

Per Serving: Calories: 409; Fat: 12g; Saturated Fat: 6g; Sodium: 399mg; Cholesterol: 193mg; Carbs: 50g; Fiber: 2g; Sugar: 11g; Protein: 23g

Eat the Rainbow Veggie Scramble

SERVES 2 / PREP TIME: 12 MINUTES / COOK TIME: 30 MINUTES

The variety of vegetables in this scramble offers a wide spectrum of vitamins and minerals, in addition to plenty of fiber. To top it off, protein from the eggs and carbohydrates from the potatoes make this a well-rounded rainbow of a meal.

2 tablespoons avocado oil, divided

8 baby potatoes (any color), cut in quarters

½ medium onion, diced

1 large carrot, shredded

1 medium red bell pepper, seeded and diced

1 tablespoon smoked paprika

Salt

Freshly ground black pepper

1 cup fresh spinach

4 eggs

1. Heat a large pan over medium heat and pour in 1 tablespoon avocado oil. When the oil is warm, add the potatoes. Cook 12–15 minutes, stirring occasionally, until potatoes are soft and slightly golden.

2. Add the remaining 1 tablespoon avocado oil, onion, carrot, bell pepper, paprika, and a pinch of salt and pepper to the pan. Cook 8 to 10 minutes, or until veggies are soft, stirring occasionally. Add the spinach and sauté until wilted, about 2 minutes.

3. In a medium bowl, whisk the eggs until well mixed. Add the eggs to the pan and scramble 5 minutes, or until cooked through.

4. Serve immediately or store covered in the refrigerator for up to three days.

COST HACK: Replace fresh vegetables with frozen mixed vegetables to save money and time. Frozen vegetables are just as nutritious as fresh because they are picked at the peak of the season and packaged immediately after harvesting.

Per Serving: Calories: 777; Fat: 24g; Saturated Fat: 5g; Sodium: 282mg; Cholesterol: 327mg; Carbs: 120g; Fiber: 20g; Sugar: 15g; Protein: 25g

Veggie Fried Rice

SERVES 2 / PREP TIME: 30 TO 50 MINUTES / COOK TIME: 20 MINUTES

Much healthier than the average fried rice, but just as satisfying, this meal includes one cup of vegetables Per Serving: and is packed with two of our favorite metabolism-boosting foods: eggs and spinach. Coconut aminos are made from coconut blossom nectar that is fermented and blended with salt; the sauce has a salty and sweet taste. The flavor is almost identical to soy sauce with less than half the amount of sodium, making this a great alternative. Most grocery stores stock coconut aminos, or they can be purchased online, but tamari or low-sodium soy sauce can be used as alternatives.

1 tablespoon avocado oil

1 cup frozen mixed vegetables (such as carrots, peas, green beans), thawed

1 cup fresh spinach

1 cup cooked brown rice

4 eggs

2 tablespoons coconut aminos

½ teaspoon red pepper flakes

1 teaspoon sesame seeds

1. Heat a large pan over medium heat. Pour in 1 tablespoon of avocado oil and the mixed veggies, spinach, and rice. Stir-fry 10 to 15 minutes, or until the rice is slightly browned and crispy.

2. Crack the eggs directly into the pan with the rice mixture and stir until the eggs are thoroughly cooked.

3. Add the coconut aminos, red pepper flakes, and sesame seeds, and stir to combine. Serve immediately.

VARIATION: You can use any leftover cooked vegetables you have on hand. If you're using fresh vegetables, cook them right in the pan before adding the rice.

Per Serving: Calories: 276; Fat: 17g; Saturated Fat: 4g; Sodium: 184mg; Cholesterol: 327mg; Carbs: 17g; Fiber: 5g; Sugar: 4g; Protein: 14g

Artichoke Turmeric Shakshuka

SERVES 4 / PREP TIME: 10 MINUTES / COOK TIME: 20 MINUTES

Shakshuka is a Mediterranean breakfast dish in which eggs are poached in a tomato sauce. This version is loaded with vegetables to bump up the fiber content and offer different flavors that will please the palate. It's amazingly simple and great to serve at a brunch gathering with a small piece of toasted whole-wheat bread on the side of each plate. Artichokes are high in vitamins C and K, and offer a unique texture and flavor. Feel free to add more fresh vegetables, such as spinach or arugula, and top the dish with a soft cheese, such as goat cheese.

2 tablespoons extra-virgin olive oil

1 small onion, thinly sliced

1 red bell pepper, seeded and thinly sliced

1 tablespoon ground turmeric

½ (12-ounce) jar low-salt marinara sauce

1 (12-ounce) jar artichoke hearts, drained and quartered

4 eggs

Salt

Freshly ground black pepper

1. Preheat the oven to 375°F.

2. Heat the olive oil in a medium ovenproof skillet (preferably cast iron) over medium-high heat. Add the onion, bell pepper, and turmeric, and sauté until softened, about 5 minutes. Lower the heat and add the marinara sauce and artichoke hearts. Mix to combine.

3. Crack the eggs into the sauce and season with salt and pepper.

4. Transfer the pan to the oven and bake 15 to 20 minutes, until the egg whites are firm but the yolks are slightly runny.

INGREDIENT TIP: Marinara sauce from a jar can be loaded with sugar and salt, so look for one with as little sugar as possible and fewer than 260mg of sodium per serving.

Per Serving: Calories: 199; Fat: 12g; Saturated Fat: 2g; Sodium: 196mg; Cholesterol: 164mg; Carbs: 18g; Fiber: 6g; Sugar: 6g; Protein: 10g

Avocado Spinach Breakfast Burrito

SERVES 4 / PREP TIME: 10 MINUTES / COOK TIME: 10 MINUTES

A warm, fresh, and filling breakfast burrito will start your day on the right foot. This recipe includes several metabolism-boosting ingredients and healthy fats, all served on a low-carb tortilla (we like the ones from La Tortilla Factory). If you can't find Vidalia onions, just use regular yellow or white onions.

Avocado oil spray

1 medium Vidalia onion, diced

½ teaspoon red pepper flakes

8 eggs

4 cups fresh spinach

4 (100-calorie) whole-wheat or gluten-free tortillas

2 medium avocados, sliced

1. Heat a sauté pan or skillet over medium heat and spray with avocado oil for 3 to 4 seconds. Add the onions and red pepper flakes and sauté until translucent, about 5 minutes.

2. While onions are cooking, beat the eggs in a large mixing bowl until well mixed.

3. Add the spinach to the cooked onions and sauté until wilted, 1 to 2 minutes. Add the beaten eggs to the pan and scramble by gently mixing with a wooden spoon as they cook. When the eggs are solid, remove the pan from the heat.

4. Spoon a quarter of the mixture onto each tortilla and top with avocado slices. Fold over at the top and bottom and roll into a burrito.

PREPARATION TIP: For an on-the-go option, lay a piece of foil on the countertop with a piece of paper towel on top of the foil. Put the finished burrito on top of the paper towel and roll it up in foil.

Per Serving: Calories: 384; Fat: 25g; Saturated Fat: 5g; Sodium: 431mg; Cholesterol: 327mg; Carbs: 27g; Fiber: 9g; Sugar: 3g; Protein: 18g

Beet and Goat Cheese Frittata with Arugula Salad

SERVES 4 / PREP TIME: 1 HOUR / COOK TIME: 20 MINUTES

Simple but rich in flavor, this creamy frittata is filled with healthy proteins. Sweet beets and tangy goat cheese are a flavor combination made in food heaven. Metabolism-boosting beets aid in detoxifying the liver and add a refreshing pop of color to this dish.

1 teaspoon avocado oil

8 eggs

½ cup plain low-fat Greek yogurt

½ teaspoon crushed red pepper flakes

Salt

Freshly ground black pepper

4 cooked beets, cut into ¼-inch slices

1 tablespoon minced fresh dill

4 ounces goat cheese, crumbled

2 cups arugula

Fresh lemon juice

1. Preheat the oven to 400° F and place a rack in the middle of the oven. Grease a medium baking dish with the avocado oil.

2. In a medium bowl, whisk together the eggs, Greek yogurt, red pepper flakes, and a pinch of salt and pepper. Pour into the baking dish and scatter the sliced beets, dill, and goat cheese evenly in the egg mixture. Bake for 18 to 20 minutes, or until the eggs set.

3. Serve immediately, or cover and store for up to three days in the refrigerator. Right before serving, squeeze the lemon juice over the arugula and season with salt and pepper. Place the salad on top of the frittata.

PREPARATION TIP: To save time, search the refrigerated section in the produce aisle of your grocery store for precooked beets. Use caution when working with beets, as their red juices can stain hands, clothing, countertops, and cutting boards.

Per Serving: Calories: 334; Fat: 20g; Saturated Fat: 10g; Sodium: 358mg; Cholesterol: 345mg; Carbs: 14g; Fiber: 2g; Sugar: 11g; Protein: 25g

Spicy Chickpeas and Eggs over Arugula

SERVES 4 / PREP TIME: 6 MINUTES / COOK TIME: 10 MINUTES

Eggs and chickpeas are packed with protein and fiber, which will leave you feeling full but energized. Paprika, chili powder, and red pepper flakes are metabolism-boosting spices that add both flavor and heat to this dish. Adjust the heat level up or down as you like. If you can't find Vidalia onions, just use regular yellow or white onions.

Avocado oil spray

½ Vidalia onion, diced

1 (15-ounce) can no-salt-added chickpeas, drained and rinsed

2 tablespoons smoked paprika

2 tablespoons chili powder

½ teaspoon red pepper flakes

8 eggs

2 cups fresh arugula

1. Heat a sauté pan or skillet over medium heat and spray with avocado oil for 3 to 4 seconds. Add the onions and sauté until translucent. Add the chickpeas, smoked paprika, chili powder, and red pepper flakes to the pan. Mash the chickpeas with a potato masher or fork until they resemble ground meat. Sauté until golden brown and crispy, about 5 minutes.

2. In a large bowl, beat the eggs until well mixed. Add the egg mixture to the chickpeas and scramble with a wooden spoon as they cook. When the eggs are solid, remove the pan from the heat.

3. Serve the egg mixture over a bed of arugula.

INGREDIENT TIPS: To avoid BPAs (epoxy resins that are used to coat the insides of some cans), purchase cans labeled "BPA-free" or cook your own dried beans instead. Your beans will be free of all additives. Cook up a big batch on the weekend, and use a pressure cooker to speed up the cooking time.

Per Serving: Calories: 267; Fat: 13g; Saturated Fat: 3g; Sodium: 170mg; Cholesterol: 327mg; Carbs: 23g; Fiber: 8g; Sugar: 5g; Protein: 18g

Loaded Hash Brown Vegetable Frittata Cups

SERVES 4 (3 PER SERVING) / PREP TIME: 12 MINUTES / COOK TIME: 30 MINUTES

This dish is an amazing grab-and-go meal for your busy mornings. Hearty and well rounded, it is packed with numerous metabolism-boosting foods, including eggs, red pepper, turmeric, and spinach. Turmeric is a bright yellow spice with an earthy aroma. It is one of our metabolism-boosting favorites and is known for its detoxifying properties, as well as its anti-inflammatory and cancer-fighting characteristics.

Nonstick cooking spray

1 (12-ounce) bag frozen shredded potatoes

8 eggs

Salt

Freshly ground black pepper

1 cup arugula

½ white onion, finely diced

1 medium red bell pepper, seeded and finely chopped

½ teaspoon red pepper flakes

1 teaspoon ground turmeric

1. Preheat the oven to 450° F and place a rack in the middle of the oven. Lightly grease a 12-cup muffin tin with nonstick cooking spray.

2. Divide the frozen shredded potatoes among the 12 muffin cups and bake for 10 minutes.

3. While the potatoes are cooking, whisk the eggs in a large bowl until well mixed. Season with salt and pepper. Add the arugula, onion, red bell pepper, red pepper flakes, and turmeric to the egg mixture and stir until evenly distributed.

4. Carefully take the pan out of the oven and press on the potatoes with a measuring cup or spoon to compact them. Pour the egg mixture evenly into each cooked potato cup and bake 20 minutes, or until the eggs are set.

VARIATION: If you can't find frozen shredded potatoes at your local market, try frozen diced potatoes or sweet potato noodles. Replace the arugula with other greens, such as baby kale, spinach, or Swiss chard.

Per Serving: Calories: 492; Fat: 28g; Saturated Fat: 5g; Sodium: 976mg; Cholesterol: 327mg; Carbs: 45g; Fiber: 6g; Sugar: 3g; Protein: 14g

Deconstructed Salmon Eggs Benedict

SERVES 2 / PREP TIME: 5 MINUTES / COOK TIME: 8 MINUTES

Vitamin D is naturally found in very few foods, and salmon is one of them! Vitamin D aids your body's immune system in functioning properly, and also helps you absorb dietary calcium. When you buy canned salmon, look for the words "Alaskan wild caught" and "purse seine fishing technique," which tells you it has been sustainably caught.

1 teaspoon avocado oil

4 eggs

2 whole-wheat English muffins

1 (6-ounce) can salmon, drained

2 tablespoons store-bought chimichurri sauce, plus more for drizzling

1 cup fresh arugula

2 thin slices red onion, cut in half

4 thin slices tomato

1. Heat a medium nonstick skillet over medium-high heat and pour in the oil. When the oil is hot, crack in 2 eggs. After 1 minute, or when the egg whites are set, use a spatula to gently flip them over. Let the eggs cook for 1 to 2 more minutes, or until the egg whites are set and the yolks are still runny. Remove from pan and repeat with the other 2 eggs, so all the eggs are cooked over-easy. Set aside until muffins are ready to be assembled.

2. While the eggs are cooking, split and toast the English muffins.

3. In a medium bowl, mix the salmon and 2 tablespoons of chimichurri sauce.

4. Top each English muffin half with ¼ cup of arugula, ½ slice of onion, and 1 slice of tomato, then carefully slide on 1 cooked egg. Top each with a quarter of the salmon mixture.

5. Drizzle each egg with additional chimichurri sauce. Serve immediately.

VARIATION TIP: Instead of the chimichurri sauce, substitute whatever you have on hand. Some delicious possibilities include sun-dried tomato pesto, basil pesto, and salsa verde.

Per Serving: Calories: 492; Fat: 24g; Saturated Fat: 5g; Sodium: 769mg; Cholesterol: 396mg; Carbs: 31g; Fiber: 3g; Sugar: 5g; Protein: 37g

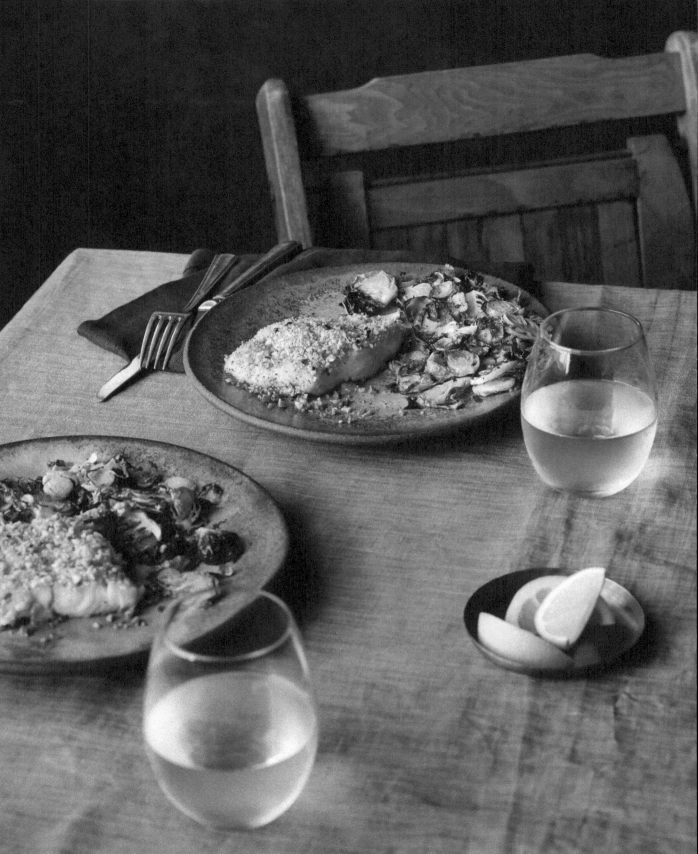

CHAPTER 4

Fish and Seafood

Lemony Halibut

SERVES 4 / PREP TIME: 5 MINUTES / COOK TIME: 10 MINUTES

Halibut is a lean fish with mild, sweet-tasting white flesh, large flakes, and a firm but tender texture. Even if you're not a fish lover, we really think you'll love this recipe. Fish cooks quickly, so pay attention to the cooking time. It's done when the fish becomes opaque and flakes easily with a fork.

4 (6-ounce) halibut steaks

Zest of 2 lemons

¼ teaspoon red pepper flakes

Salt

Freshly ground black pepper

2 tablespoons extra-virgin olive oil

1. Season the halibut steaks all over with lemon zest, red pepper flakes, salt, and pepper.

2. Heat a medium pan over medium-high heat and pour in the olive oil. When the oil is hot and shimmering, add the halibut. Let it cook undisturbed for 3 to 4 minutes, then flip and cook 3 to 4 more minutes.

3. Serve with lemon slices from the zested lemons.

PREPARATION TIP: Use a fine grater to zest the lemon, or use a potato peeler to peel the rind away from the white pith, then cut it into thin strips.

Per Serving: Calories: 238; Fat: 11g; Saturated Fat: 1g; Sodium: 128mg; Cholesterol: 49mg; Carbs: 0g; Fiber: 0g; Sugar: 0g; Protein: 35g

Seared Ahi Tuna

SERVES 4 / PREP TIME: 10 MINUTES / COOK TIME: 10 MINUTES

Tuna is high in omega-3 fatty acids that will leave you feeling fuller longer, especially when combined with fiber. For a complete meal, enjoy with some brown rice and Zesty Broccoli with Garlic and Red Pepper Flakes (page 124).

¼ cup sesame seeds

½ teaspoon red pepper flakes

½ teaspoon ground ginger

4 (6-ounce) ahi tuna fillets

Salt

Freshly ground black pepper

2 tablespoons extra-virgin olive oil

1. Mix the sesame seeds, red pepper flakes, and ginger on a plate.
2. Season the tuna fillets with salt and pepper, then press both sides into the sesame mixture to coat.
3. Heat a medium nonstick pan over medium heat and pour in the oil. When the oil is hot and shimmering, add the tuna fillets and cook about 2 minutes on each side.
4. Remove from pan and let sit 1 to 2 minutes before serving.

INGREDIENT TIP: To create contrast and make the dish more visually appealing, use a mixture of black and golden sesame seeds.

Per Serving: Calories: 323; Fat: 15g; Saturated Fat: 2g; Sodium: 100mg; Cholesterol: 90mg; Carbs: 8g; Fiber: 2g; Sugar: 0g; Protein: 39g

Lime-Baked Snapper

SERVES 4 / PREP TIME: 15 MINUTES / COOK TIME: 15 MINUTES

Red snapper is a low-calorie, low-fat source of protein that is rich in selenium, vitamin A, potassium, and omega-3 fatty acids. This recipe actually works well with all kinds of fish, shellfish, and even chicken breasts. Make it a meal by serving with Lime Quinoa (page 134) and steamed asparagus.

4 limes, zested and sliced

2 cloves garlic, finely chopped

1 shallot, finely chopped

½ teaspoon red pepper flakes

2 tablespoons avocado oil

4 (6-ounce) snapper fillets

Salt

Freshly ground black pepper

1. Preheat the oven to 400° F. Line a large baking sheet with foil.

2. In a small bowl, mix the lime zest, garlic, shallot, red pepper flakes, and oil.

3. Season the fish with a pinch of salt and pepper. Rub the lime mixture all over the fish until evenly distributed.

4. Spread the lime slices over the baking sheet and top with the seasoned fish.

5. Bake for 10 to 15 minutes, or until the fish is cooked through.

Per Serving: Calories: 231; Fat: 4g; Saturated Fat: 0g; Sodium: 138mg; Cholesterol: 79mg; Carbs: 1g; Fiber: 0g; Sugar: 0g; Protein: 44g

Blackened Tilapia

SERVES 4 / PREP TIME: 5 MINUTES / COOK TIME: 15 MINUTES

Tilapia is a low-mercury fish that is safe even for pregnant women to eat. It is also a lean source of protein and high in several vitamins and minerals, including selenium, vitamin B_{12}, niacin, and potassium. Make it a meal by serving with Tropical Mango Slaw (page 121) and wild rice.

4 (6-ounce) tilapia fillets

Salt

1 teaspoon smoked paprika

½ teaspoon cayenne pepper

¼ teaspoon ground ginger

¼ teaspoon dried oregano

¼ teaspoon fennel seeds

⅛ teaspoon ground cloves

¼ teaspoon black pepper

2 tablespoons avocado oil

1. Season the tilapia with a pinch of salt.

2. In a small bowl, mix paprika, cayenne pepper, ground ginger, oregano, fennel seeds, ground cloves, and black pepper. Sprinkle evenly over both sides of the fish.

3. Heat a large nonstick pan over medium-high heat. Pour in the avocado oil and when it is hot and shimmering, place the fillets in the pan. Cook 5 to 6 minutes on each side, or until cooked through.

Per Serving: Calories: 206; Fat: 9g; Saturated Fat: 2g; Sodium: 100mg; Cholesterol: 83mg; Carbs: 1g; Fiber: 0g; Sugar: 0g; Protein: 32g

Miso-Glazed Cod

SERVES 4 / PREP TIME: 15 MINUTES / COOK TIME: 15 MINUTES

Miso is a protein-rich paste made from fermented soybeans. It comes in several varieties: white, which is slightly sweet; yellow, which is earthy and mild; and red, which is the saltiest. You can find it at most grocery stores and Asian food markets in the refrigerated section; it will keep in the refrigerator for a long time. As a fermented food, miso provides the good bacteria that help your gut stay healthy and happy. Gut health is known to be linked to overall mental and physical wellness. Serve with brown rice and a simple salad to make a meal.

¼ cup white miso paste

1 tablespoons rice wine vinegar

1 teaspoon honey

1 teaspoon peeled and minced fresh ginger

1 clove garlic, finely minced

2 teaspoons toasted sesame oil

4 (6-ounce) skinless cod fillets

Freshly ground black pepper

1. Preheat the oven to 450°F. Line a large baking sheet with foil.

2. In a medium bowl, whisk together the miso, rice wine vinegar, honey, ginger, garlic, and sesame oil.

3. Place the fish on the lined baking sheet and season both sides with a pinch of pepper. Pour the miso glaze evenly over the fish.

4. Bake for 15 minutes, or until the fish is firm and easily flakes.

PREPARATION TIP: For an even better flavor, let the fish marinate in the miso mixture for 15 to 30 minutes at room temperature before putting it in the oven.

Per Serving: Calories: 174; Fat: 3g; Saturated Fat: 0g; Sodium: 630mg; Cholesterol: 60mg; Carbs: 8g; Fiber: 0g; Sugar: 5g; Protein: 32g

Almond-Crusted Cod Fillets

SERVES 4 / PREP TIME: 10 MINUTES / COOK TIME: 20 MINUTES

Cod is a great source of selenium, a mineral that is critical for proper thyroid function. Combined with slivered almonds and Parmesan cheese, this dish is a true crowd-pleaser. Serve with brown rice and Crispy Roasted Brussels Sprouts with Balsamic Drizzle (page 125).

½ cup slivered almonds, finely chopped

¼ cup grated Parmesan cheese

1 lemon, zested and cut into wedges

1 teaspoon garlic powder

½ teaspoon red pepper flakes

4 (6-ounce) skinless cod fillets

Salt

Freshly ground black pepper

1. Preheat the oven to 400° F. Line a large baking sheet with foil or parchment paper.

2. In a medium bowl, mix the chopped almonds, Parmesan cheese, lemon zest, garlic powder, and red pepper flakes.

3. Place the fish on the baking sheet and season with a pinch of salt and pepper. Spread the almond mixture evenly on top of each fillet.

4. Bake 15 to 20 minutes, or until the fish is cooked through and flakes easily with a fork. Serve with lemon wedges on the side.

VARIATION: Substitute a different white fish, such as tilapia, flounder, or snapper. Be sure to reduce the cooking time if you are using thinner fillets; check for doneness at 7 to 10 minutes.

Per Serving: Calories: 229; Fat: 9g; Saturated Fat: 2g; Sodium: 224mg; Cholesterol: 65mg; Carbs: 3g; Fiber: 2g; Sugar: 1g; Protein: 35g

Panko and Walnut-Crusted Rockfish

SERVES 2 / PREP TIME: 10 MINUTES / COOK TIME: 16 MINUTES

Whole-wheat panko contributes fiber and gives a pleasing crunch to each bite of lightly seasoned rockfish. Pair with Crispy Roasted Multicolored Baby Potatoes (page 127) and Roasted Asparagus (page 118) to complete and round off the meal. Cook both in the same oven at the same temperature—you can even place the potatoes and asparagus on the same baking sheet.

1 tablespoon extra-virgin olive oil

½ cup whole-wheat panko

¼ cup walnuts, chopped

½ teaspoon red pepper flakes

Zest of 1 lemon

2 (6-ounce) rockfish fillets

Salt

Freshly ground black pepper

1. Preheat the oven to 425° F. Coat the bottom of a medium baking dish with the oil.

2. In a small bowl, mix the whole-wheat panko, chopped walnuts, red pepper flakes, and lemon zest.

3. Season the fillets with salt and pepper. Place the fish in the baking dish and cover with the panko mixture.

4. Bake for 14 to 16 minutes, until the fish is baked through and the panko is golden and crisp.

INGREDIENT TIP: Rockfish actually refers to several varieties of Pacific white-fleshed fish that are mild in flavor. It is also referred to as rock cod or Pacific snapper. Feel free to purchase either of these varieties, or your favorite white fish if you cannot find rockfish at your local market.

Per Serving: Calories: 418; Fat: 21g; Saturated Fat: 2g; Sodium: 253mg; Cholesterol: 80mg; Carbs: 13g; Fiber: 3g; Sugar: 0g; Protein: 18g

Jamaican Mahi-Mahi

SERVES 4 / PREP TIME: 10 MINUTES / COOK TIME: 15 MINUTES

This unique recipe is perfect on a warm summer day. Plus, your body will love the metabolism-boosting effects of the yummy spices! You can use store-bought jerk seasoning mix to save on time but still produce the same great flavor. Unless you are familiar with the flavors of jerk, though, choose the mild one; jerk seasoning can be *very* spicy.

1 teaspoon celery salt

1 teaspoon onion powder

1 teaspoon garlic powder

1 teaspoon sweet paprika

½ teaspoon ground coriander

½ teaspoon dried thyme

4 (6-ounce) mahi-mahi fillets

Salt

Freshly ground black pepper

2 tablespoons avocado oil

1. In a small bowl, mix the celery salt, onion powder, garlic powder, paprika, coriander, and thyme.

2. Season the mahi-mahi fillets with salt and pepper. Sprinkle the spice mixture evenly over the fillets.

3. Heat a medium nonstick pan over medium heat and pour in the avocado oil. When the oil is hot and shimmering, add the fillets. Cook 4 to 5 minutes on each side, or until thoroughly cooked.

PREPARATION TIP: Put the spices in large zip-top bag and mix to combine. Place the fish in the same zip-top bag, close, and shake to coat the fish. This makes for even seasoning distribution and easy cleanup.

Per Serving: Calories: 203; Fat: 7g; Saturated Fat: 1g; Sodium: 185mg; Cholesterol: 60mg; Carbs: 1g; Fiber: 0g; Sugar: 1g; Protein: 32g

Chimichurri Baked Salmon

SERVES 4 / PREP TIME: 5 MINUTES / COOK TIME: 15 MINUTES

We love this recipe because, besides the salt and pepper, it uses only two ingredients! Salmon is such a delicious fish; it doesn't need to be prepared in a fancy way. Chimichurri is a green sauce from Argentina that is traditionally made with parsley, garlic, oregano, and olive oil. This sauce has become so popular that you can buy it in jars in the store. But if you want to make your own, there's a recipe for it in Chimichurri Pork Tenderloin (page 108).

4 (6-ounce) skinless salmon fillets

Salt

Freshly ground black pepper

¼ cup store-bought chimichurri sauce

1. Preheat the oven 425° F. Line a large baking sheet with foil.
2. Season the fillets on both sides with a pinch of salt and pepper. Place them on the baking sheet and pour the chimichurri evenly over the salmon. Rub to coat.
3. Bake for 10 to 15 minutes, or until the salmon is thoroughly cooked.

VARIATION: On the same baking sheet, add broccoli or cauliflower and cover in chimichurri. To make a complete balanced meal, serve it with brown rice or a small baked potato.

Per Serving: Calories: 360; Fat: 24g; Saturated Fat: 4g; Sodium: 231mg; Cholesterol: 104mg; Carbs: 1g; Fiber: 0g; Sugar: 0g; Protein: 33g

Sesame-Crusted Salmon

SERVES 4 / PREP TIME: 5 MINUTES / COOK TIME: 10 MINUTES

Vitamin-rich sesame seeds make for a crunchy coating and contribute a pleasant nutty flavor. Enjoy with Lime Quinoa (page 134) and Tropical Mango Slaw (page 121) to freshen the meal and enjoy for any lunch or dinner.

¼ cup sesame seeds

½ teaspoon red pepper flakes

4 (6-ounce) skinless salmon fillets

Salt

Freshly ground black pepper

2 tablespoons extra-virgin olive oil

1. Mix the sesame seeds and red pepper flakes on a plate.

2. Season the salmon fillets with salt and pepper. Press the fillets into the spice mixture on both sides to coat.

3. Heat medium nonstick pan over medium heat and pour in the olive oil. When the oil is hot and shimmering, add the salmon fillets. Cook 3 to 4 minutes on each side, until cooked through.

COST HACK: You can use any leftovers in the Deconstructed Salmon Eggs Benedict (page 71) for a variation on that dish, as well as saving time and money.

Per Serving: Calories: 412; Fat: 30g; Saturated Fat: 5g; Sodium: 137mg; Cholesterol: 97mg; Carbs: 2g; Fiber: 1g; Sugar: 0g; Protein: 35g

Salmon Cakes

SERVES 4 / PREP TIME: 15 MINUTES / COOK TIME: 20 MINUTES

You will absolutely love our nutritious spin on a traditional salmon cake. Avocado mayonnaise is mayo made with healthy avocado oil. Find it in the supermarket or at health food stores. And bonus: Canned salmon contains a good amount of omega-3 fatty acids. This dish is easy to prepare and doesn't need to be deep-fried to taste good. Serve it with arugula salad, lemon wedges, and brown rice.

1 (14.75-ounce) can plus 1 (5-ounce) can skinless, boneless pink salmon

¼ cup whole-wheat panko

2 tablespoons grainy mustard

2 tablespoons avocado mayonnaise

1½ tablespoons chopped fresh dill

1 tablespoon finely chopped shallot

2 teaspoons chopped capers

1. Preheat the oven to 400° F. Line a large baking sheet with parchment paper.

2. Drain the salmon and flake it into a large bowl. Stir in the panko, mustard, mayonnaise, dill, shallots, and capers until well combined.

3. Form into 8 patties, about ⅓ cup each. Let rest 5 minutes, then place the patties on the baking sheet. Make sure they are evenly spaced.

4. Bake 20 minutes, or until the patties are slightly golden and warmed through.

PREPARATION TIP: You can pan sear the salmon patties on the stovetop in 1 tablespoon of extra-virgin olive oil, 4 minutes per side, before baking to create a crust. If you do, cut the baking time in half.

Per Serving: Calories: 271; Fat: 10g; Saturated Fat: 3g; Sodium: 725mg; Cholesterol: 48mg; Carbs: 7g; Fiber: 1g; Sugar: 0g; Protein: 32g

Italian-Style Salmon in Foil Packs

SERVES 4 / PREP TIME: 20 MINUTES / COOK TIME: 10 MINUTES

Turn any casual barbecue into a gourmet food experience with our Italian grilled salmon. As a bonus, the foil packs help keep your grill mess-free. If you don't have a grill, though, you can bake this recipe at 450°F for 10 to 15 minutes or cook the foil packets on a stovetop grill pan over medium-high heat for 10 minutes.

4 (6-ounce) skinless salmon fillets

1 tablespoon chopped fresh rosemary

Salt

Freshly ground black pepper

2 lemons, sliced

4 teaspoons capers

½ cup Marsala wine (optional)

1. Preheat your grill to medium-high heat.

2. Cut 4 large pieces of foil. Place 1 salmon fillet on each piece of foil. Season each fillet with rosemary and a pinch of salt and pepper. Top each salmon with 2 to 3 lemon slices, 1 teaspoon of capers, and 2 tablespoons of Marsala wine (if using).

3. Wrap up the salmon tightly into foil packets. Grill on the hot grill 10 minutes, or until the fish is thoroughly cooked.

Per Serving: Calories: 303; Fat: 18g; Saturated Fat: 4g; Sodium: 222mg; Cholesterol: 97mg; Carbs: 1g; Fiber: 0g; Sugar: 0g; Protein: 33g

Grilled Salmon with Cilantro Yogurt Sauce

SERVES 4 / PREP TIME: 10 MINUTES / COOK TIME: 15 MINUTES

One of our favorite recipes, this salmon dish can be served cold over a salad or hot alongside your favorite grain. Don't skimp on the jalapeño pepper; it might be a little spicy, but remember it helps give your metabolism a temporary boost. Serve with brown rice and Fresh Corn Salad Speckled with Cilantro (page 122).

1 tablespoon avocado oil

Zest and juice of 1 lime

1 teaspoon honey

Salt

Freshly ground black pepper

1 jalapeño pepper, seeded and finely chopped

1 clove garlic, finely chopped

1 cup finely chopped fresh cilantro

½ cup plain low-fat Greek yogurt

4 (6-ounce) skinless salmon fillets

Olive oil spray

1. Preheat the grill to medium heat. Or preheat the oven to 400° F.

2. In a medium bowl, mix the avocado oil, lime zest, lime juice, honey, and a pinch of salt and pepper until well combined. Add the jalapeño pepper, garlic, cilantro, and Greek yogurt, and mix until well combined. Set aside.

3. Season the salmon fillets with a pinch of salt and pepper. Spray the grill or coat a medium baking pan with olive oil spray.

4. Grill the salmon about 4 minutes on each side, or until cooked through and firm to the touch. Or bake in the oven for 15 minutes.

5. Serve with the sauce spooned over the top.

PREPARATION TIP: To get the most juice out of the lime, roll it on the countertop or microwave it for 5 to 10 seconds.

Per Serving: Calories: 361; Fat: 22g; Saturated Fat: 4g; Sodium: 153mg; Cholesterol: 98mg; Carbs: 4g; Fiber: 0g; Sugar: 3g; Protein: 36g

Golden Baked Sea Bass in Parchment Packets

SERVES 4 / PREP TIME: 15 MINUTES / COOK TIME: 15 MINUTES

The skins of citrus fruits are bursting with vitamin C and antioxidants. You can add orange, lemon, or lime zest to our other seafood recipes as well for added nutrition and a burst of bright flavor. Serve with brown rice and Roasted Asparagus (page 118).

1 teaspoon ground turmeric

1 orange, zested and sliced

½ teaspoon black pepper

½ teaspoon dried thyme

1 teaspoon honey

1 tablespoon extra-virgin olive oil

4 (6-ounce) sea bass fillets

1. Preheat the oven to 450° F. Cut 4 large pieces of parchment paper.

2. In a small bowl, mix the turmeric, orange zest, pepper, thyme, honey, and olive oil. Brush each fillet with the turmeric paste.

3. Put 2 to 3 slices of orange on each piece of parchment paper. Top each with 1 piece of seasoned, brushed fish. Fold the parchment over, creating a packet, and fold over the edges to create a seal.

4. Put the packets on a large baking sheet and bake 10 to 12 minutes. Turn the oven off and let the fish sit in the oven 1 minute longer. The pouch should have puffed up.

5. Remove from oven, let the pouch cool 1 to 2 minutes, then open, being careful of the steam inside.

VARIATION: You can make this recipe with any white fish fillets, such as cod, tilapia, or mahi-mahi.

Per Serving: Calories: 352; Fat: 23g; Saturated Fat: 5g; Sodium: 189mg; Cholesterol: 69mg; Carbs: 9g; Fiber: 2g; Sugar: 6g; Protein: 29g

Quick Curried Fish Stew

SERVES 4 / PREP TIME: 10 MINUTES / COOK TIME: 20 MINUTES

Curry is a blend of spices used in Indian cuisine and throughout Asia. It may help control blood sugar and assist your liver in detoxifying heavy metals, such as lead and mercury. Serve this dish with Coconut Brown Rice (page 135) and a side salad.

2 tablespoons olive oil

1 onion, finely chopped

2 cloves garlic, finely chopped

1-inch piece fresh ginger, peeled and finely chopped

Salt

Freshly ground black pepper

4 tablespoons curry powder

1 (14.5-ounce) can diced tomatoes

½ cup light coconut milk

1 pound cod fillets or other firm white fish, cut into bite-size chunks

1. Pour the oil in a large nonstick pan over medium heat. Add the onion, garlic, ginger, and a pinch of salt and pepper. Sauté until the onion is translucent, about 5 minutes. Add the curry powder and sauté for 2 minutes, until the curry is fragrant and well mixed with the onion.

2. Add the diced tomatoes and coconut milk. Mix to combine and bring to a simmer.

3. Season the fish with a pinch of salt and pepper and add to the pan. Cook until fish is firm and cooked through, about 8 minutes.

STORAGE TIP: Place leftover rice and fish stew in an airtight glass container for an easy lunch the next day. It will keep in the refrigerator up to three days.

Per Serving: Calories: 219; Fat: 11g; Saturated Fat: 3g; Sodium: 126mg; Cholesterol: 55mg; Carbs: 12g; Fiber: 4g; Sugar: 4g; Protein: 23g

Shrimp Ceviche

SERVES 4 / PREP TIME: 15 MINUTES, PLUS 30 MINUTES TO MARINATE

Ceviche is a Latin American dish made with fish or seafood that is cured in fresh lemon or lime juice. This cooling dish is naturally flavored with a wide array of vegetables. Pair the ceviche with corn tortillas for an additional source of carbohydrates to round out the meal.

1 pound cooked shrimp, peeled, deveined, and coarsely chopped

Juice of 3 large limes

1 jalapeño pepper, seeded and chopped

½ white onion, finely chopped

1 medium cucumber, finely chopped

1 pint cherry tomatoes, halved

1 avocado, chopped

¼ cup chopped fresh cilantro

Salt

1. In a large bowl, mix shrimp, lime juice, jalapeño, onion, cucumber, cherry tomatoes, avocado, and cilantro with a generous pinch of salt.

2. Let stand for 20 to 30 minutes so the flavors blend.

PREPARATION TIP: If you're starting with raw shrimp, cook them in boiling water for about 3 minutes, or until pink. Make sure the shrimp is cooked before adding it to the rest of the ingredients.

Per Serving: Calories: 250; Fat: 9g; Saturated Fat: 2g; Sodium: 327mg; Cholesterol: 239mg; Carbs: 16g; Fiber: 5g; Sugar: 5g; Protein: 28g

Garlic Fennel Shrimp

SERVES 4 / PREP TIME: 10 MINUTES / COOK TIME: 10 MINUTES

Shrimp is an extremely low-calorie source of protein, which can help you stay full while losing weight. Pair it with fennel, which is high in both fiber and flavor. Enjoy this meal for lunch or dinner, and feel free to serve it with more vegetables.

2 tablespoons extra-virgin olive oil, divided

1 bulb fennel, sliced

5 cloves garlic, finely chopped

¼ teaspoon red pepper flakes

1 pound fresh shrimp, shelled and deveined

Salt

Freshly ground black pepper

1. Heat a medium pan over medium-high heat and pour in 1 tablespoon of olive oil. When the oil is hot and shimmering, add the sliced fennel and sauté until soft, about 8 minutes. Add the garlic and red pepper flakes.

2. Pat the shrimp dry with paper towels and season with a pinch of salt and pepper. Add 1 more tablespoon of olive oil to the pan, then add the shrimp.

3. Cook the shrimp for 2 minutes on each side, until pink.

PREPARATION TIP: To cut a fennel bulb, simply cut it in half from the root end to the top. Peel away the outer layer and cut into thin slices.

Per Serving: Calories: 174; Fat: 7g; Saturated Fat: 1g; Sodium: 210mg; Cholesterol: 160mg; Carbs: 8g; Fiber: 2g; Sugar: 0g; Protein: 22g

Garlicky Shrimp Scampi

SERVES 4 / PREP TIME: 10 MINUTES / COOK TIME: 12 MINUTES

A healthy spin on a traditional Italian dish, our shrimp scampi is enjoyed over fresh zucchini instead of white pasta. Refined carbohydrates like pasta can wreak havoc on your metabolism by spiking blood sugar levels.

4 tablespoons extra-virgin olive oil, divided

24 unpeeled raw jumbo shrimp (about 2 pounds), shelled

Salt

Freshly ground black pepper

1 shallot, finely chopped

2 packages zucchini noodles (fresh or frozen)

Zest and juice of 1 lemon

½ teaspoon red pepper flakes

2 tablespoons chopped fresh thyme

4 cloves garlic, minced

1. Heat large nonstick pan over medium heat and pour in 2 tablespoons of olive oil.

2. Season the shrimp with a pinch of salt and pepper. When the oil shimmers, add the shrimp to the pan and sear on both sides until pink, about 2 to 3 minutes per side. Remove from the pan and set aside.

3. To same skillet add 2 more tablespoons of olive oil, then the shallot and zucchini noodles. Season with lemon zest, red pepper flakes, thyme, garlic, and a pinch of salt and pepper. Cook until softened, 2 to 3 minutes. Take the pan off the heat and add the shrimp back to the pan. Squeeze the lemon juice over the shrimp and serve.

PREPARATION TIP: Zest the lemon before cutting it for the juice, to make it easier to zest the whole fruit. To zest a lemon, use a fine grater or a potato peeler to remove the zest and slice very thin into strips, avoiding the white pith.

PREPARATION TIP: To make your own zucchini noodles use a handheld vegetable spiralizer cutter. Cut both ends off two zucchinis. Place one tip of the zucchini in the spiralizer and twist in one smooth motion, applying slight pressure so that the noodles are formed. Repeat with second zucchini and use immediately.

Per Serving: Calories: 345; Fat: 15g; Saturated Fat: 2g; Sodium: 342mg; Cholesterol: 320mg; Carbs: 13g; Fiber: 3g; Sugar: 4g; Protein: 45g

Sumac and Cayenne Spiced Scallops

SERVES 4 / PREP TIME: 2 MINUTES / COOK TIME: 10 MINUTES

Scallops offer high amounts of protein and are a fantastic no-hassle seafood. A hint of heat from cayenne pepper, tanginess from sumac, and a sprinkle of salt and pepper bring out the natural scallop flavor. Sumac is a purple Middle Eastern spice. It has a tangy flavor that helps enhance the taste of meat and vegetable dishes. Fresh lemon zest is an easy substitute for sumac.

12 large fresh scallops

Salt

Freshly ground black pepper

1 tablespoon ground sumac

½ teaspoon cayenne pepper

2 tablespoons avocado oil

1. Season the scallops with a pinch of salt and pepper. Sprinkle the sumac and cayenne pepper evenly over each scallop.

2. Heat a large nonstick pan over medium-high heat. Pour in the avocado oil and when it is hot and shimmers, place the scallops in the pan. They should rest evenly on the bottom; if the pan is overcrowded, cook them in batches.

3. Cook 3 to 4 minutes on each side, or until cooked through.

COST HACK: If you use frozen scallops, be sure to thaw them according to the package directions. Frozen scallops have the same nutritional value as fresh ones and often cost less.

Per Serving: Calories: 162; Fat: 8g; Saturated Fat: 1g; Sodium: 221mg; Cholesterol: 37mg; Carbs: 3g; Fiber: 0g; Sugar: 0g; Protein: 19g

Clam, Shrimp, and Potato Bake

SERVES 4 / PREP TIME: 15 MINUTES / COOK TIME: 15 MINUTES

Perfect for a large gathering, our grilled clam bake is a healthy entrée your friends and family can enjoy! Pair this with a simple salad or any vegetable for a healthy meal.

¼ cup extra-virgin olive oil

3 cloves garlic, minced

2 tablespoons chopped fresh flat-leaf parsley

1 tablespoon chopped fresh dill

Zest of 1 lemon

2 tablespoons Old Bay Seasoning, divided

1 pound baby yellow potatoes

2 ears corn, shucked and each cut into 4 pieces

24 unpeeled raw jumbo shrimp (about 2 pounds), shelled

24 littleneck clams in shells, scrubbed

2 lemons, each cut into 4 wedges

2 tablespoons chopped fresh chives

1. Preheat the grill to medium heat. Or preheat the oven to 400° F. Cut 8 (12-inch-square) pieces of heavy-duty aluminum foil.

2. In a medium bowl, mix together the olive oil, garlic, parsley, dill, lemon zest, and 1 tablespoon of Old Bay Seasoning.

3. Poke each potato with a fork and place on a plate. Microwave on high until the potatoes are tender and a knife can be inserted easily in the center, about 5 minutes.

4. Place 4 squares of the foil in a single layer on work surface. Place 3 potatoes and 2 pieces of corn on each foil sheet. To each, add 6 shrimp and 6 clams. Top each with 2 lemon wedges and 1 tablespoon of the oil mixture, and sprinkle with 1 teaspoon of Old Bay. Top each with a foil square, and crimp all sides to seal tightly.

5. If you're using a grill, close the lid and grill the packets until the shrimp are done and the clams open, 8 to 10 minutes. If you're using an oven, bake 12 to 15 minutes until the clams open and shrimp are pink. Discard any clams that do not open. Sprinkle with fresh chives just before serving.

COST HACK: Buy frozen shrimp and thaw under cool running water. Most fresh shrimp have been frozen and thawed anyway.

Per Serving: Calories: 498; Fat: 16g; Saturated Fat: 3g; Sodium: 827mg; Cholesterol: 383mg; Carbs: 38g; Fiber: 6g; Sugar: 4g; Protein: 54g

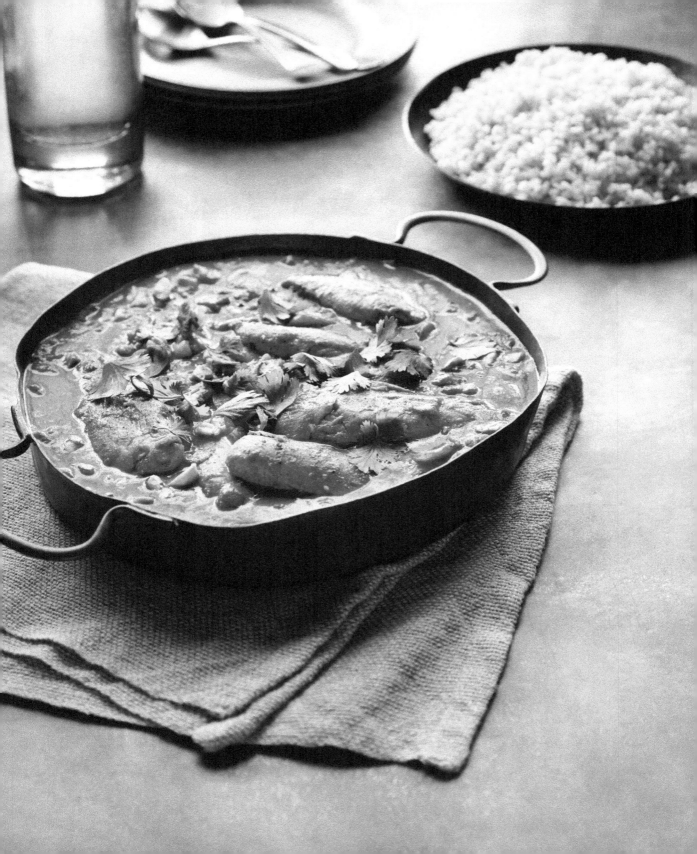

CHAPTER 5

Poultry and Meat

Rosemary Lemon Chicken

SERVES 4 / PREP TIME: 10 MINUTES / COOK TIME: 12 MINUTES

This recipe requires very few ingredients and has a delicious, refreshing flavor. Cubing the chicken breast makes it perfect to use on salads. Store leftovers in the refrigerator and add to a bowl of arugula or mixed greens for a quick and healthy lunch.

4 boneless, skinless chicken breasts, cubed

1 tablespoon finely chopped fresh rosemary

2 cloves garlic, finely chopped

Zest of 1 lemon

Salt

Freshly ground black pepper

2 tablespoons extra-virgin olive oil

1. Rub the chicken with rosemary, garlic, lemon zest, and a pinch of salt and pepper.

2. Heat a nonstick skillet on medium-high heat. Add the olive oil, then the chicken cubes. Cook 10 to 12 minutes, tossing so all sides cook evenly, until the chicken is cooked thoroughly.

VARIATION: Try this dish with other fresh herbs, such as thyme, tarragon, or dill.

Per Serving: Calories: 185; Fat: 9g; Saturated Fat: 1g; Sodium: 114mg; Cholesterol: 65mg; Carbs: 1g; Fiber: 0g; Sugar: 0g; Protein: 27g

Green Chili Baked Chicken

SERVES 4 / PREP TIME: 5 MINUTES / COOK TIME: 30 MINUTES

Green chilies contain large amounts of vitamin A and are surprisingly high in fiber. This dish is fantastic on a weeknight because of how little preparation time it needs. We suggest serving the chicken with our Lime Quinoa (page 134) and steamed broccoli for a complete meal.

4 small boneless, skinless chicken breasts (about 1 pound total)

2 (4-ounce) cans mild chopped green chilies

1 teaspoon chili powder

Salt

Freshly ground black pepper

1. Preheat the oven to 375° F.
2. In a large baking dish, combine chicken, green chilies, chili powder, salt, and pepper. Mix to coat evenly.
3. Bake 25 to 30 minutes, or until the chicken is cooked thoroughly.

VARIATION: You can make this recipe with a pork loin roast as well. Insert a meat thermometer in the center of the pork loin and roast until the internal temperature reaches 145°F, about 30 minutes.

Per Serving: Calories: 134; Fat: 2g; Saturated Fat: 0g; Sodium: 345mg; Cholesterol: 65mg; Carbs: 3g; Fiber: 1g; Sugar: 0g; Protein: 27g

Chili Lime Chicken

SERVES 4 / PREP TIME: 10 MINUTES / COOK TIME: 7 MINUTES

Lime zest is packed with vitamin C and is actually more nutritionally dense than the citrus flesh. Together with a dash of chili powder, this chicken has just the right amount of heat and will spice up any meal.

4 boneless, skinless chicken breasts, thinly sliced

Salt

Freshly ground black pepper

Zest of 2 limes

2 cloves garlic, finely chopped

1 shallot, finely chopped

½ teaspoon chili powder

2 tablespoons avocado oil

1. Season the chicken with salt and pepper.
2. In a small bowl, mix the lime zest, garlic, shallot, chili powder, and avocado oil. Rub each piece of chicken with the mixture, coating all sides.
3. Heat a nonstick skillet on medium-high heat. Put the seasoned chicken in the skillet. Cook 5 to 7 minutes, tossing to ensure all sides cook evenly, until the chicken is cooked thoroughly.

VARIATION: Substitute a firm-fleshed white fish for the chicken. Shorten the cooking time, though, because fish tends to cook more quickly than chicken.

Per Serving: Calories: 187; Fat: 9g; Saturated Fat: 1g; Sodium: 118mg; Cholesterol: 65mg; Carbs: 1g; Fiber: 0g; Sugar: 0g; Protein: 27g

Greek Lemony Oregano Chicken

SERVES 4 / PREP TIME: 5 MINUTES / COOK TIME: 20 MINUTES

This recipe features fresh oregano, which is high in antioxidants and also has antibacterial properties. It has a history of being used to treat a variety of illnesses, including urinary tract infections, respiratory tract infections, and gastrointestinal disorders.

4 whole boneless, skinless chicken breasts

1 tablespoon finely chopped fresh oregano

2 cloves garlic, finely chopped

Zest of 1 lemon

Salt

Freshly ground black pepper

2 to 3 tablespoons extra-virgin olive oil

1 tablespoon lemon juice

1. Rub the chicken with the oregano, garlic, lemon zest, and a pinch of salt and pepper.

2. Heat a nonstick skillet on medium-high heat. Pour in the olive oil and then add the chicken. Cook the chicken 15 to 20 minutes, flipping halfway through, until it reaches an internal temperature of 165° F and is cooked thoroughly.

3. When chicken is cooked and ready to be removed from the skillet, drizzle with the lemon juice.

VARIATION: Bake this chicken in a baking dish at 375°F under a bed of seasoned freshly sliced onions, zucchini, and Kalamata olives.

Per Serving: Calories: 187; Fat: 9g; Saturated Fat: 1g; Sodium: 115mg; Cholesterol: 65mg; Carbs: 1g; Fiber: 1g; Sugar: 0g; Protein: 27g

Fragrant Sumac Chicken

SERVES 4 / PREP TIME: 12 MINUTES / COOK TIME: 10 MINUTES

Sumac, lemon juice, and thyme give this chicken breast a refreshingly tangy flavor while also boosting health. Ingredients such as sumac and thyme developed a reputation for medicinal properties in ancient cultures. Sumac is known to be good for heart health and thyme for boosting immunity.

4 boneless, skinless chicken breasts, sliced into thin strips

Salt

Freshly ground black pepper

1 tablespoon ground sumac

Juice of 1 lemon

1 tablespoon finely chopped fresh thyme

4 cloves garlic, finely chopped

2 to 3 tablespoons extra-virgin olive oil

1. Season the chicken with salt and pepper.

2. In a small bowl, mix the sumac, lemon juice, thyme, and garlic. Rub each piece of chicken, coating all sides.

3. Heat a nonstick skillet on medium-high heat. Pour in the olive oil, then add the chicken. Cook 3 to 5 minutes per side, until the chicken is thoroughly cooked.

Per Serving: Calories: 191; Fat: 9g; Saturated Fat: 1g; Sodium: 77mg; Cholesterol: 65mg; Carbs: 3g; Fiber: 1g; Sugar: 1g; Protein: 27g

Sun-Dried Tomato Roasted Chicken

SERVES 4 / PREP TIME: 6 MINUTES / COOK TIME: 35 MINUTES

This recipe uses only four simple ingredients and is the absolute best for when you are in a rush to get dinner on the table. It features sun-dried tomato pesto, which provides a good source of healthy fat from olive oil, and has a tangier flavor than traditional basil pesto.

4 boneless, skinless chicken breasts

¼ cup store-bought sun-dried tomato pesto, drained of some excess oil

Salt

Freshly ground black pepper

1. Preheat the oven to 425°F.
2. In a large baking dish, combine the chicken, sun-dried tomato pesto, and a pinch of salt and pepper. Rub the chicken until evenly coated.
3. Bake 30 to 35 minutes, or until the chicken is cooked thoroughly.

COST HACK: Often, store-bought pesto contains an excess amount of oil. Be sure to drain some oil into an airtight container so you can use it later. This will condense the pesto sauce for this dish. Use the leftover pesto oil to sauté your favorite vegetables.

Per Serving: Calories: 143; Fat: 3g; Saturated Fat: 0g; Sodium: 261mg; Cholesterol: 65mg; Carbs: 2g; Fiber: 0g; Sugar: 1g; Protein: 27g

Crispy Parmesan Rosemary Chicken Tenders

SERVES 4 / PREP TIME: 10 MINUTES / COOK TIME: 20 MINUTES

Who doesn't love a good chicken tender? These are a great, healthy spin on regular chicken tenders, using a lighter and more nutritious whole-wheat panko rather than a dense breading. Not to mention the use of the metabolism-boosting herb rosemary.

1 pound chicken tenders

Salt

Freshly ground black pepper

1 ½ cups whole-wheat panko

¼ cup shredded Parmesan cheese

1 teaspoon dried rosemary

2 eggs

1. Preheat the oven to 400° F. Line a large baking sheet with parchment paper.

2. Season the chicken tenders with a pinch of salt and pepper. In a shallow bowl, mix together the panko, Parmesan, and rosemary. In a separate shallow bowl, beat the eggs. Working with one tender at a time, dredge in the egg, followed by the Parmesan panko.

3. Place the tenders on the lined baking sheet. Bake for 20 minutes, or until lightly golden and cooked through.

PREPARATION TIP: Use two paper plates for the breading instead of shallow bowls. This saves time on cleanup.

Per Serving: Calories: 259; Fat: 5g; Saturated Fat: 2g; Sodium: 262mg; Cholesterol: 152mg; Carbs: 17g; Fiber: 2g; Sugar: 0g; Protein: 34g

Miso-Glazed Chicken

SERVES 4 / PREP TIME: 8 MINUTES / COOK TIME: 35 MINUTES

This dish is good for your gut. Miso is a fermented food rich in B vitamins that promotes the growth of healthy gut bacteria. In addition, freshly grated ginger and garlic are great anti-inflammatory foods that reduce bloating. Marinate the chicken overnight in the refrigerator to deepen the miso flavor.

4 (4- to 6-ounce) boneless, skinless chicken breasts

¼ cup white miso paste

1 tablespoon rice wine vinegar

1 teaspoon honey

1 teaspoon grated fresh ginger

1 clove garlic, grated

2 teaspoons toasted sesame oil

1. Preheat the oven to 400° F. Line a large baking sheet with foil.

2. In a large bowl, whisk the miso, vinegar, honey, ginger, garlic, and sesame oil. Mix well, then add the chicken and rub to coat.

3. Place the chicken on the lined baking sheet, and pour any miso glaze from the bowl evenly on each chicken breast.

4. Bake 30 to 35 minutes, or until the chicken is cooked thoroughly.

PREPARATION TIP: Place all ingredients in a large zip-top plastic bag and shake until the chicken is well coated. This makes for easier cleanup.

Per Serving: Calories: 183; Fat: 5g; Saturated Fat: 1g; Sodium: 1975mg; Cholesterol: 65mg; Carbs: 6g; Fiber: 1g; Sugar: 4g; Protein: 27g

Cashew Chicken Curry in a Hurry

SERVES 4 / PREP TIME: 12 MINUTES / COOK TIME: 25 MINUTES

This well-rounded recipe incorporates protein and healthy fats into one delicious curry. In addition, cashews contain a compound called zeaxanthin, which is a type of beta-carotene that is beneficial for eye health. Add spinach for a vegetable component and serve with Coconut Brown Rice (page 135).

1 tablespoon extra-virgin olive oil

1 medium white onion, diced

3 cloves garlic, finely chopped

2-inch piece fresh ginger, peeled and finely chopped or grated

¼ cup curry powder

1 pound chicken tenders

Salt

Freshly ground black pepper

1 (14.5-ounce) can low-sodium diced tomatoes

2 tablespoons plain low-fat Greek yogurt

2 tablespoons finely chopped raw unsalted cashews

1. Heat a large pot on medium-high heat and pour in the oil. Sauté the onion, garlic, ginger, and curry powder until the onions begin to soften and become translucent, about 5 minutes.

2. Add the chicken to the pan and season with a pinch of salt and pepper. Cook until the chicken is almost done, 10 to 15 minutes. Add the tomatoes and cook until the chicken is thoroughly done, about 5 minutes more.

3. Take the pan off the heat and stir in the Greek yogurt and cashews.

VARIATION: Garnish with chopped fresh cilantro to enhance and balance the curry flavor.

Per Serving: Calories: 272; Fat: 8g; Saturated Fat: 1g; Sodium: 171mg; Cholesterol: 67mg; Carbs: 13g; Fiber: 3g; Sugar: 6g; Protein: 38g

Oven-Baked Chicken Shawarma

SERVES 4 / PREP TIME: 8 MINUTES / COOK TIME: 30 MINUTES

Shawarma hails from the Middle East, and is traditionally thin slices of meat cooked slowly on a large rotisserie spit. This at-home version is quicker and easier, and is also seasoned with a variety of aromatic spices—including cumin, which contains high amounts of iron and has long been used to treat indigestion. Serve your shawarma the traditional way: with Tzatziki Yogurt Sauce with Whole-Wheat Pita (page 145) and Marinated Cucumber and Tomato Salad (page 146).

4 cloves garlic, grated

1 tablespoon smoked paprika

2 teaspoons ground cumin

½ teaspoon red pepper flakes

Juice of 1 lemon

1 tablespoon extra-virgin olive oil

1 teaspoon honey

1½ pounds whole boneless, skinless chicken breasts

Salt

Freshly ground black pepper

1. Preheat the oven to 425° F. Line a large baking sheet with foil.

2. In a medium bowl, combine the garlic, smoked paprika, cumin, red pepper flakes, lemon juice, oil, and honey.

3. Season the chicken with a pinch of salt and pepper and toss with the spice mixture to coat evenly.

4. Arrange the chicken in an even layer on the lined baking sheet. Bake for 30 minutes, or until chicken is cooked thoroughly.

VARIATION: Substitute thinly sliced beef for the chicken. Bake in the oven for 12 minutes, or until it's cooked to your liking.

Per Serving: Calories: 232; Fat: 6g; Saturated Fat: 1g; Sodium: 157mg; Cholesterol: 98mg; Carbs: 4g; Fiber: 1g; Sugar: 2g; Protein: 40g

Sheet Pan French Onion Chicken

SERVES 4 / PREP TIME: 5 MINUTES / COOK TIME: 35 MINUTES

A simple mixture of fresh herbs and sweet yellow onions produces a delicious flavor every time. Thyme, in particular, is high in antibacterial properties and is commonly used to alleviate the irritations of sore throats and bronchitis. Serve this dish with Crispy Roasted Multicolored Baby Potatoes (page 127) and a side salad.

½ cup chicken stock

1 tablespoon Worcestershire sauce

2 onions, thinly sliced

1 tablespoon olive oil

½ teaspoon red pepper flakes

2 tablespoons fresh thyme leaves

1 tablespoon chopped fresh sage

1 pound chicken tenders

Salt

Freshly ground black pepper

1. Preheat the oven to 425° F.

2. Pour the chicken stock into a large baking dish. Add the Worcestershire sauce, onions, oil, red pepper flakes, thyme, and sage. Mix to combine.

3. Season the chicken with a pinch of salt and pepper. Place it in the baking dish on top of the onion mixture.

4. Bake 30 to 35 minutes, or until the chicken is cooked thoroughly.

VARIATION: You can make this recipe in the slow cooker. Simply place all ingredients in the cooker the night before and store in the refrigerator. Turn on the slow cooker at noon and the recipe will be done in 6 hours on low heat, just in time for dinner. For a faster cooking time, set the slow cooker on high for 4 hours.

Per Serving: Calories: 190; Fat: 6g; Saturated Fat: 1g; Sodium: 176mg; Cholesterol: 66mg; Carbs: 8g; Fiber: 2g; Sugar: 3g; Protein: 28g

Ground Turkey Tacos

SERVES 4 / PREP TIME: 10 MINUTES / COOK TIME: 16 MINUTES

Ground turkey is an affordable protein that has a much lower saturated fat content than ground beef. So don't give up tacos—just make your current taco recipe healthier by substituting ground turkey. Most people can't even tell the difference! Serve with corn tortillas, shredded lettuce, store-bought salsa (read the labels and watch out for added salt and sugar), and sliced avocado to make a complete meal.

1 tablespoon extra-virgin olive oil

½ medium onion, diced

2 cloves garlic, minced

1 pound lean ground turkey

2 teaspoons ground cumin

1 teaspoon chili powder

¼ teaspoon dried oregano

1 teaspoon smoked paprika

½ teaspoon salt

1. Heat a large nonstick pan over medium-high heat. Pour in the olive oil and when it shimmers, put the onions in the pan and cook 3 to 5 minutes, or until the onions are translucent. Then add the garlic and sauté 1 minute more.

2. Add the turkey, cumin, chili powder, oregano, paprika, and salt, and mix well. Break the meat up with a wooden spoon or spatula and sauté until the turkey starts to crumble and is cooked thoroughly, 7 to 10 minutes.

PREPARATION TIP: For finer taco meat crumbles, lightly press the ground turkey with a potato masher while cooking it. To make the ground turkey moister, add 1 to 2 tablespoons of water when the turkey starts to crumble, about 5 minutes after meat is added to the pan, and cook down until a sauce forms.

Per Serving: Calories: 208; Fat: 12g; Saturated Fat: 3g; Sodium: 386mg; Cholesterol: 81mg; Carbs: 3g; Fiber: 1g; Sugar: 1g; Protein: 23g

Chimichurri Pork Tenderloin

SERVES 4 / PREP TIME: 15 MINUTES, PLUS 15 MINUTES TO MARINATE / COOK TIME: 18 MINUTES

The ingredients in a chimichurri sauce bring freshness to the rich pork tenderloin. While this recipe can be prepared the day you cook the meat, marinate the tenderloin overnight in the refrigerator for a stronger and deeper flavor.

1 (1-pound) boneless pork tenderloin

Salt

Freshly ground black pepper

4 cloves garlic, grated

1 jalapeño pepper, seeded and finely chopped

¼ cup red wine vinegar

½ cup finely chopped fresh flat-leaf parsley

½ cup finely chopped fresh cilantro

Juice of 3 limes

½ cup extra-virgin olive oil

1. Preheat the grill over medium-high heat. Or preheat the oven to 450°F and line a large baking sheet with foil.

2. Season the pork tenderloin with a pinch of salt and pepper.

3. In a medium glass jar, mix the garlic, jalapeño, vinegar, parsley, cilantro, lime juice, olive oil, and a heavy pinch of salt and pepper.

4. Reserve ½ cup of the chimichurri sauce to serve with the cooked pork. Pour the rest into a large zip-top bag, add the pork, and mix well. Set aside to marinate 10 to 15 minutes.

5. Oil the grill and cook the pork on the hottest part of the grill for 4 to 6 minutes per side, or until cooked thoroughly. If using the oven, place the pork on the baking sheet and cook for 18 minutes, or until a meat thermometer reads an internal temperature of 145°F.

6. Allow the pork to rest 5 minutes before slicing. Spoon 1 to 2 tablespoons of chimichurri sauce over each serving.

COST HACK: Double up the chimichurri recipe and save it in an airtight glass jar to pour over eggs, other proteins, or roasted vegetables. It will keep up to 5 days in the refrigerator.

Per Serving: Calories: 384; Fat: 31g; Saturated Fat: 6g; Sodium: 103mg; Cholesterol: 74mg; Carbs: 5g; Fiber: 1g; Sugar: 1g; Protein: 25g

Coffee-Rubbed Pork Tenderloin

SERVES 4 / PREP TIME: 8 MINUTES / COOK TIME: 25 MINUTES

Although we discourage coffee or any caffeine during the four-week metabolism reset, this recipe is a nice little teaser! There's not enough coffee in it to really make a difference. And the unique flavors are sure to wow your friends and family. Serve with Crispy Roasted Multicolored Baby Potatoes (page 127) and a side salad.

2 tablespoons ground coffee

1 tablespoon brown sugar

2 teaspoons smoked paprika

½ teaspoon ground ginger

½ teaspoon onion powder

½ teaspoon garlic powder

1 (1-pound) boneless pork tenderloin

Salt

Freshly ground black pepper

1. Preheat the oven to 400° F. Line a baking sheet with foil.
2. In a small bowl, mix the coffee grounds, brown sugar, paprika, ginger, onion powder, and garlic powder.
3. Season the pork tenderloin with a pinch of salt and pepper and place in a zip-top bag with the coffee mixture. Shake to coat.
4. Place the pork on the lined baking sheet and tent with another piece of foil. Bake 10 minutes, then remove the foil and continue to cook 10 to 15 minutes more, or until the pork is cooked thoroughly.

VARIATION: You can cook this dish on the grill over medium-high heat for 15 to 20 minutes.

Per Serving: Calories: 163; Fat: 6g; Saturated Fat: 2g; Sodium: 97mg; Cholesterol: 64mg; Carbs: 4g; Fiber: 1g; Sugar: 2g; Protein: 24g

Pan-Seared Pork Chops with Mushroom Sherry Sauce

SERVES 4 / PREP TIME: 10 MINUTES / COOK TIME: 20 MINUTES

This is an elegant dish. Mushrooms are rich in B vitamins and add a wonderful richness to any meal. Sherry brings another depth of flavor to the meal and contains beneficial phenolic compounds. Serve these chops with brown rice or baked potatoes and steamed vegetables.

4 boneless, thick pork chops, fat trimmed

Salt

Freshly ground black pepper

1 teaspoon sweet paprika

2 tablespoons extra-virgin olive oil

1 white onion, sliced

12 cremini mushrooms, stems removed

1 tablespoon finely chopped fresh thyme

½ cup sherry

1. Season the pork chops with salt, pepper, and paprika.

2. Heat a nonstick skillet on medium-high heat. Pour in the olive oil, then add the pork chops. Cook 4 to 5 minutes per side. Transfer the pork to a plate and tent with foil to keep warm.

3. In same pan, add the sliced onions and cook until translucent, about 5 minutes. Add the mushrooms and cook 1 to 2 minutes more. Then add a hearty pinch of pepper, and the thyme and sherry. Lower the heat and cook until the sauce thickens, 2 to 3 minutes. Serve over the pork.

VARIATION: If you don't like mushrooms, swap them out for fresh zucchini. Or just add both!

Per Serving: Calories: 313; Fat: 20g; Saturated Fat: 6g; Sodium: 483mg; Cholesterol: 55mg; Carbs: 6g; Fiber: 1g; Sugar: 2g; Protein: 27g

Herb-Baked Steak Bites

SERVES 4 / PREP TIME: 10 MINUTES / COOK TIME: 20 MINUTES

Herbs such as rosemary and thyme complement steak's natural flavors. Cooking with organic grass-fed beef helps to boost your metabolism, because it is more nutrient-dense than conventionally raised beef. It tastes better, too.

1 tablespoon finely chopped fresh rosemary

1 tablespoon finely chopped fresh thyme

2 cloves garlic, minced or grated

½ teaspoon black pepper

1 tablespoon extra-virgin olive oil

1 pound grass-fed beef sirloin, cubed

Salt

1. Preheat the oven to 425°F. Line a baking sheet with foil.

2. In a large zip-top bag or bowl, mix the rosemary, thyme, garlic, pepper, oil, beef, and a pinch of salt. Shake to mix evenly.

3. Spread the beef out on the lined baking sheet with foil. Bake 15 to 20 minutes, or until the steak is cooked thoroughly.

VARIATION: You can make this recipe with other cuts of beef, such as filet mignon or top round. It also makes for great grilling. Be sure to oil the grill to prevent the seasonings from sticking.

Per Serving: Calories: 144; Fat: 7g; Saturated Fat: 3g; Sodium: 87mg; Cholesterol: 67mg; Carbs: 2g; Fiber: 1g; Sugar: 0g; Protein: 20g

Beef Stir-Fry

SERVES 4 / PREP TIME: 10 MINUTES / COOK TIME: 12 MINUTES

This is a super simple stir-fry that is perfect after a long day at work. Coconut aminos are a great substitute for soy sauce if you are trying to avoid gluten or soy. Serve with steamed broccoli and brown rice to make a complete meal.

1 pound grass-fed flank steak, thinly sliced

½ teaspoon ground turmeric

Salt

Freshly ground black pepper

2 tablespoons coconut aminos

4 tablespoons water

1-inch piece fresh ginger, peeled and finely grated

4 cloves garlic, finely chopped

½ teaspoon red pepper flakes

1 tablespoon cornstarch

2 to 3 tablespoons avocado oil

1. Season the steak with turmeric and a pinch of salt and pepper.

2. In a small bowl, mix the coconut aminos, water, ginger, garlic, red pepper flakes, and cornstarch.

3. Heat a nonstick skillet on medium-high heat and pour in the oil. Add the steak to the hot skillet. Stir-fry 5 to 7 minutes, until the steak is cooked.

4. Stir in the sauce mixture. Simmer 2 to 4 minutes, or until the sauce has thickened.

VARIATION: Swap thinly sliced chicken for the steak. Brown the chicken in a medium skillet 4 minutes on each side and simmer in the sauce mixture for 2 to 4 minutes, or until the sauce has thickened.

Per Serving: Calories: 333; Fat: 24g; Saturated Fat: 0g; Sodium: 49mg; Cholesterol: 40mg; Carbs: 5g; Fiber: 2g; Sugar: 0g; Protein: 24g

Sheet Pan Steak Fajitas

SERVES 4 / PREP TIME: 15 MINUTES / COOK TIME: 25 MINUTES

Chili powder and cayenne pepper are rich in antioxidants and high in vitamins C, E, and B_6. Both promote digestion by stimulating salivary glands and gastric juices, boosting metabolism and encouraging detoxification in the body. Serve this savory dish with corn tortillas and fresh sliced avocado.

1 pound grass-fed flank steak, thinly sliced

½ teaspoon cayenne pepper

1 large red onion, sliced

1 green bell pepper, seeded and sliced

1 red bell pepper, seeded and sliced

1 zucchini, sliced

2 tablespoons chili powder

Salt

Freshly ground black pepper

2 tablespoons avocado oil

1. Preheat the oven to 425° F. Line two baking sheets with foil.

2. Season the flank steak with cayenne pepper and place on a baking sheet. Place the onion, bell peppers, and zucchini on the other baking sheet.

3. Season the contents of each baking sheet with 1 tablespoon of chili powder, a pinch of salt and pepper, and 1 tablespoon of avocado oil.

4. Bake 20 to 25 minutes, or until the beef is cooked thoroughly and the vegetables are softened.

VARIATION: Squeezing fresh lime juice over the cooked beef and vegetables will bring a nice balance to this dish. You can also use store-bought MSG-free taco seasoning rather than chili powder and cayenne.

Per Serving: Calories: 309; Fat: 14g; Saturated Fat: 6g; Sodium: 180mg; Cholesterol: 81mg; Carbs: 12g; Fiber: 4g; Sugar: 4g; Protein: 33g

Mediterranean Spiced Beef Meatballs

SERVES 4 / PREP TIME: 10 MINUTES / COOK TIME: 30 MINUTES

Seasoned with a variety of metabolism-boosting spices, these meatballs are perfect in wraps, salads, and bowls. In addition, this is a fun dish to prepare with family or friends by having them help roll the meatballs.

1 tablespoon ground cumin

1 tablespoon ground coriander

1 tablespoon cinnamon

1 teaspoon salt

1 teaspoon pepper

1 pound grass-fed lean ground beef

1 small onion, grated

2 cloves garlic, grated

1. Preheat the oven to 375° F. Line a large baking sheet with foil.

2. In a medium bowl, mix cumin, coriander, cinnamon, salt, pepper, beef, onion, and garlic together with your hands until everything is well-incorporated. Roll into about 16 meatballs the size of golf balls.

3. Evenly space the meatballs on the baking sheet. Bake for 25 to 30 minutes.

VARIATION: You can make this recipe with ground turkey. Bake for 20 minutes, or until the internal temperature reaches 165°F.

Per Serving: Calories: 220; Fat: 10g; Saturated Fat: 5g; Sodium: 560mg; Cholesterol: 75mg; Carbs: 5g; Fiber: 2g; Sugar: 1g; Protein: 24g

Spiced Beef Kebabs

SERVES 4 / PREP TIME: 10 MINUTES, PLUS 15 MINUTES TO MARINATE / COOK TIME: 8 MINUTES

Using Greek yogurt in this marinade will seal the moisture into the flank steak. Smoked paprika and turmeric are high in antioxidants and help lower inflammation in the body. These kebabs pair well with our Roasted Sesame Sweet Potatoes (page 128).

1 cup low-fat plain Greek yogurt

1-inch piece fresh ginger, peeled, finely grated

2 cloves garlic, finely chopped

½ teaspoon ground turmeric

1 teaspoon smoked paprika

¼ teaspoon cinnamon

Juice of 1 lemon

1 pound grass-fed flank steak, thinly sliced against the grain into 1-inch strips

Avocado oil

1. Preheat a grill pan or heavy skillet over medium-high heat.

2. In a large mixing bowl, combine Greek yogurt, ginger, garlic, turmeric, paprika, cinnamon, and lemon juice. Add the sliced steak and mix to coat. Set aside to marinate 10 to 15 minutes.

3. Thread the beef strips on metal or wooden skewers.

4. Oil the grill grates or skillet and place the beef skewers on the pan. Cook 3 to 4 minutes per side, or until the steak is cooked thoroughly.

PREPARATION TIP: Instead of mixing the marinade in a bowl, use a large zip-top bag to save cleanup time.

Per Serving: Calories: 241; Fat: 11g; Saturated Fat: 3g; Sodium: 94mg; Cholesterol: 61mg; Carbs: 4g; Fiber: 0g; Sugar: 2g; Protein: 31g

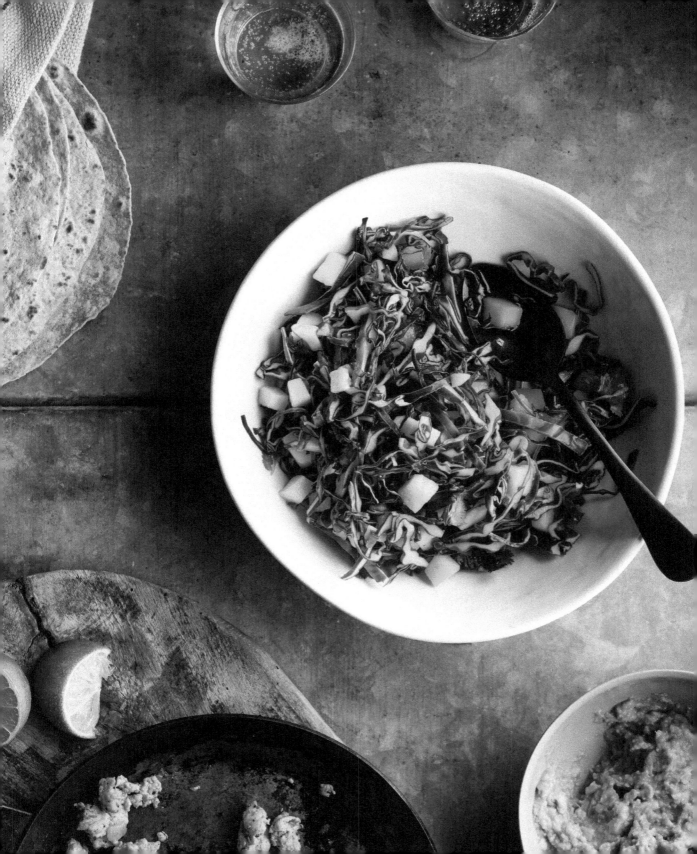

CHAPTER 6

Vegetables and Grains

TROPICAL MANGO SLAW, PAGE 121

Roasted Asparagus

SERVES 4 / PREP TIME: 10 MINUTES / COOK TIME: 20 MINUTES

This recipe uses only four ingredients and requires minimal prep time. Asparagus, known for being high in folate content, has a sweet yet savory flavor and doesn't need anything other than a pinch of salt and a drizzle of olive oil.

1 pound fresh asparagus spears

1 tablespoon extra-virgin olive oil

Salt

Freshly ground black pepper

1. Preheat the oven to 425° F. Line a rimmed baking sheet with foil.

2. Check to see how much to cut off the bottoms of the asparagus by taking one spear and bending it until the bottom snaps. (It ranges from 1 to 2 inches.) Bunch up the ends and cut them all at the same length where the bottom snapped.

3. On the baking sheet, toss the trimmed asparagus spears with olive oil and a pinch of salt and pepper.

4. Roast 20 minutes, or until browned and crispy.

VARIATION: Add additional spices you have on hand for variety. Try red pepper flakes, fresh chopped thyme, or fresh chopped rosemary. Be sure to use the same herbs in all the dishes when preparing a meal. This pulls the flavors together and complements the meal.

Per Serving Calories: 53; Fat: 4g; Saturated Fat: 1g; Sodium: 41mg; Cholesterol: 0mg; Carbs: 4g; Fiber: 3g; Sugar: 3g; Protein: 2g

Parmesan Roasted Carrots

SERVES 2 / PREP TIME: 10 MINUTES / COOK TIME: 20 MINUTES

High in antioxidants, carrots get their orange color from beta-carotene and are loaded with vitamin A. Savory Parmesan cheese complements the natural sweetness of carrots and creates a vegetable side dish that lightens rich meat dishes.

1 pound fresh carrots, peeled and sliced

¼ teaspoon dried thyme or 1 teaspoon chopped fresh thyme

½ teaspoon red pepper flakes

1 tablespoon extra-virgin olive oil

Salt

Freshly ground black pepper

3 tablespoons grated Parmesan cheese

1. Preheat the oven to 450° F. Line a rimmed baking sheet with parchment paper.
2. Place the carrots on the baking sheet and toss with thyme, red pepper flakes, oil, and a pinch of salt and pepper.
3. Roast until tender and slightly browned, 15 to 20 minutes. Toss with the cheese before serving.

VARIATION: Add ½ pound quartered small potatoes to the carrot dish. Be sure to add an extra tablespoon of oil to coat.

Per Serving Calories: 222; Fat: 12g; Saturated Fat: 4g; Sodium: 329mg; Cholesterol: 15mg; Carbs: 23g; Fiber: 6g; Sugar: 11g; Protein: 9g

Roasted Sesame Bok Choy

SERVES 4 / PREP TIME: 10 MINUTES / COOK TIME: 15 MINUTES

Bok choy is extremely high in antioxidants. Just one cup of this cruciferous vegetable will provide roughly 64 percent of your daily dietary need for vitamin K. If you're not a bok choy fan, you can make this recipe with any cruciferous vegetable, such as broccoli, cauliflower, or Brussels sprouts.

½ tablespoon finely grated fresh ginger

½ teaspoon red pepper flakes

1 teaspoon sesame seeds, plus extra for garnish

1 teaspoon honey

2 tablespoons coconut aminos

1 pound bok choy, halved lengthwise

Olive oil cooking spray or 1 tablespoon extra-virgin olive oil

1. Preheat the oven to 450° F. Line a rimmed baking sheet with parchment paper.

2. In a large zip-top bag or a large bowl, mix the ginger, red pepper flakes, sesame seeds, honey, and coconut aminos. Add the bok choy and toss to coat. Set aside any dressing that remains in the bowl after you remove the bok choy.

3. Place the bok choy on the baking sheet, cut side up. Spray with cooking spray or drizzle with the olive oil. Roast until tender and slightly browned, 10 to 15 minutes.

4. Drizzle with the remaining dressing and sprinkle with more sesame seeds.

Per Serving Calories: 65; Fat: 4g; Saturated Fat: 1g; Sodium: 83mg; Cholesterol: 0mg; Carbs: 6g; Fiber: 1g; Sugar: 3g; Protein: 2g

Tropical Mango Slaw

SERVES 4 / PREP TIME: 15 MINUTES, PLUS 15 MINUTES TO CHILL

Mangos are extremely high in vitamin C: Just 1 cup will provide about 70 percent of your daily recommended dietary intake. Most grocery stores carry pre-shredded purple cabbage, which offers the same nutrients as uncut cabbage. This will save time in preparing the dish. Top your Ground Turkey Tacos (page 107) with our tropical slaw.

Juice of 3 limes

1 teaspoon honey

½ teaspoon salt

4 cups finely shredded purple cabbage

1 small mango, peeled and finely diced

1 fresh jalapeño pepper, seeded and finely diced

⅓ cup finely chopped fresh cilantro

1. In a large bowl or storage container, mix the lime juice, honey, and salt. Let sit for 5 minutes so the flavors blend.

2. Add the cabbage, mango, jalapeño pepper, and cilantro and gently toss together.

3. Cover and refrigerate for at least 15 minutes and up to 48 hours.

STORAGE TIP: The longer this slaw sits, the better the taste and texture. It will keep in the refrigerator for 4 days.

Per Serving Calories: 83; Fat: 0g; Saturated Fat: 0g; Sodium: 306mg; Cholesterol: 0mg; Carbs: 21g; Fiber: 3g; Sugar: 16g; Protein: 2g

Fresh Corn Salad Speckled with Cilantro

SERVES 4 / PREP TIME: 15 MINUTES / COOK TIME: 10 MINUTES

Grilled corn, jalapeño pepper, and chili powder work together to give this salad a little heat and a hint of smokiness. Corn is a starchy whole grain that contains high amounts of vitamin C and offers a good amount of fiber, making this a nutritious option as a side dish at any picnic or barbecue.

2 tablespoons avocado oil

**Kernels cut from
4 ears fresh corn**

**1 jalapeño pepper, seeded
and finely chopped**

Salt

1 teaspoon chili powder

**½ cup chopped
fresh cilantro**

**¼ cup scallions,
thinly sliced**

Juice of 1 lime

1. Heat a large skillet over medium-high heat and pour in the avocado oil. When it is hot and shimmering, add the corn and jalapeño and a pinch of salt. Cook without stirring until the corn begins to char, 2 to 3 minutes. Stir and continue to cook 4 to 5 minutes more.

2. Add the chili powder, cilantro, scallion, and lime juice. Toss to coat the corn mixture.

3. Remove from heat immediately and enjoy.

PREPARATION TIP: If fresh corn is not in season, use thawed frozen corn kernels instead.

Per Serving Calories: 192; Fat: 9g; Saturated Fat: 1g; Sodium: 68mg; Cholesterol: 0mg; Carbs: 30g; Fiber: 5g; Sugar: 9g; Protein: 5g

Roasted Beet Citrus Salad

SERVES 4 / PREP TIME: 15 MINUTES / COOK TIME: 4 MINUTES

Beets are the star of this dish. Their rich red color and sweet, earthy flavor are full of nutrients such as folate, fiber, and potassium, not to mention phytochemicals. Pairing beets with the sweetness of oranges, creamy avocado, and a crunch from the almonds makes this dish satisfying, simple, and effortless. You can serve it immediately or store in the refrigerator for up to one day. Most grocery stores now sell precooked beets in the refrigerated produce section. Canned beets can be used as a substitute.

3 tablespoons raw unsalted almonds

1 tablespoon balsamic vinegar

2 tablespoons extra-virgin olive oil

Salt

Freshly ground black pepper

8 small cooked beets

2 oranges, segmented

1 avocado, sliced lengthwise

1. Preheat the oven to 350° F.
2. Spread almonds on a rimmed baking sheet and bake for 3 to 4 minutes, stirring halfway through. Chop coarsely and set aside.
3. Peel the beets and cut into ¼-inch slices.
4. In a small bowl, whisk together the balsamic vinegar, olive oil, and a pinch of salt and pepper.
5. In a large bowl, combine the beets and orange segments. Toss gently with the dressing. Top with sliced avocado and toasted almonds.

PREPARATION TIP: To segment the orange, trim both ends of the orange. Using a sharp paring knife, cut the peel away from the flesh, removing all the white pith. Using the knife, carefully segment the orange by slicing between the membrane and the fruit. Squeeze any extra juice over the beets.

Per Serving Calories: 290; Fat: 16g; Saturated Fat: 2g; Sodium: 196mg; Cholesterol: 0mg; Carbs: 36g; Fiber: 10g; Sugar: 25g; Protein: 6g

Zesty Broccoli with Garlic and Red Pepper Flakes

SERVES 4 / PREP TIME: 12 MINUTES / COOK TIME: 11 MINUTES

Broccoli is loaded with fiber and high in iron, potassium, and vitamin C. Seasoned with red pepper, garlic, and lemon, this dish has a classic and versatile flavor and pairs well with many different protein recipes.

1 tablespoon extra-virgin olive oil

3 cloves garlic, minced

½ teaspoon red pepper flakes

1 bunch broccoli, trimmed and cut into bite-size pieces

Zest and juice of 2 lemons

Salt

Freshly ground black pepper

1. Heat a large skillet over medium-high heat and pour in the olive oil. Add the garlic and red pepper flakes and cook for 1 minute, until fragrant and the garlic begins to brown.

2. Stir in the broccoli and cook until the broccoli is bright green, 3 to 5 minutes.

3. Add the lemon zest, juice, and a pinch of salt and pepper and continue to cook for 3 to 5 more minutes, or until the broccoli is tender.

PREPARATION TIP: Buying precut broccoli will save prep time. Frozen broccoli florets are a good substitute. Be sure to defrost the frozen broccoli before using in this recipe, following the directions on the bag.

Per Serving Calories: 79; Fat: 4g; Saturated Fat: 0g; Sodium: 81mg; Cholesterol: 0mg; Carbs: 9g; Fiber: 3g; Sugar: 3g; Protein: 4g

Crispy Roasted Brussels Sprouts with Balsamic Drizzle

SERVES 4 / PREP TIME: 12 MINUTES / COOK TIME: 25 MINUTES

Especially high in vitamin K, Brussels sprouts are also rich in fiber and can help you feel full for a long time. Additionally, the probiotics in balsamic vinegar promote digestion, making this dish not only delicious, but also good for your gut health. For extra convenience, some grocery stores carry pre-shredded Brussels sprouts; find these in the refrigerated produce section.

1 pound Brussels sprouts, thinly sliced

1 tablespoon extra-virgin olive oil

Salt

Freshly ground black pepper

½ cup balsamic vinegar

½ teaspoon red pepper flakes

3 cloves garlic, minced

1 teaspoon honey

1. Preheat the oven to 400° F. Line a rimmed baking sheet with parchment paper.

2. Spread the shredded Brussels sprouts on the baking sheet, and toss with olive oil and a pinch of salt and pepper. Roast until tender and slightly browned, 20 to 25 minutes. Stir halfway through to ensure they are evenly cooked.

3. While the Brussels sprouts are cooking, in a small saucepan, add the balsamic vinegar, red pepper flakes, garlic, and honey. Bring to a simmer over medium heat and reduce over low heat until slightly thickened, 3 to 5 minutes.

4. Drizzle the balsamic glaze over the roasted Brussels sprouts.

COST HACK: Save any leftover balsamic drizzle for up to 1 week in an airtight container in the refrigerator. It's great drizzled on other cooked vegetables or even meat recipes, such as our Coffee-Rubbed Pork Tenderloin (page 109).

Per Serving Calories: 95; Fat: 4g; Saturated Fat: 1g; Sodium: 69mg; Cholesterol: 0mg; Carbs: 13g; Fiber: 4g; Sugar: 4g; Protein: 4g

Lemon Pepper Cauliflower Steaks Topped with Panko

SERVES 4 / PREP TIME: 14 MINUTES / COOK TIME: 27 MINUTES

Cauliflower is a great low-carb, high-fiber, versatile vegetable that is used as a substitution for rice, potatoes, and even pizza crust. Here, Parmesan cheese helps meld all these flavors together and create a unique vegetable dish with a fantastic crunchy exterior.

1 large cauliflower, sliced into 1-inch steaks (about 4 steaks)

3 tablespoons extra-virgin olive oil, divided

2 teaspoons lemon pepper

1 cup whole-wheat panko

¼ cup grated Parmesan cheese

¼ cup finely chopped walnuts

½ teaspoon red pepper flakes

1. Preheat the oven to 450° F. Line a rimmed baking sheet with parchment paper.

2. Place the cauliflower steaks on the baking sheet, and drizzle each with ½ tablespoon of olive oil and ¼ teaspoon of lemon pepper. Bake 15 to 20 minutes, until the cauliflower starts to brown and soften.

3. While the cauliflower stakes are baking, in a small bowl, mix the panko, Parmesan, walnuts, 1 teaspoon lemon pepper, red pepper flakes, and 1 tablespoon olive oil.

4. Remove the baking sheet from the oven and evenly top the cauliflower steaks with the panko mixture. Return to the oven and continue to roast until the panko starts to brown, 5 to 7 minutes.

PREPARATION TIP: To prepare the cauliflower steaks, trim the inedible leaves from the bottom. Cut down the middle of the cauliflower head from top to bottom (this keeps the florets together). Do the same for each cauliflower half, providing hearty slices about 1- to 1½-inch thick. You should end up with 4 steaks.

Per Serving Calories: 229; Fat: 17g; Saturated Fat: 3g; Sodium: 132mg; Cholesterol: 5mg; Carbs: 15g; Fiber: 6g; Sugar: 5g; Protein: 8g

Crispy Roasted Multicolored Baby Potatoes

SERVES 4 / PREP TIME: 10 MINUTES / COOK TIME: 30 MINUTES

Imagine this colorful array of red, white, and even purple perfectly crisped baby potatoes alongside a juicy herb-roasted chicken breast—what could beat that? As another bonus, baby potatoes are extremely high in vitamin C and actually contain more potassium than a banana!

1 pound baby multicolored potatoes, quartered

1 tablespoon extra-virgin olive oil

½ teaspoon red pepper flakes

Salt

Freshly ground black pepper

1. Preheat the oven to 425° F. Line a rimmed baking sheet with parchment paper.

2. Place the potatoes on the baking sheet and toss with olive oil, red pepper flakes, and a pinch of salt and pepper.

3. Roast until tender and slightly browned, about 30 minutes.

VARIATION: Add root vegetables such as carrots, parsnips, and beets to the same baking dish for variety. Chop all the vegetables to a similar size so they cook evenly in the oven.

Per Serving Calories: 109; Fat: 4g; Saturated Fat: 1g; Sodium: 46mg; Cholesterol: 0mg; Carbs: 18g; Fiber: 3g; Sugar: 1g; Protein: 2g

Roasted Sesame Sweet Potatoes

SERVES 4 / PREP TIME: 6 MINUTES / COOK TIME: 25 MINUTES

There is a lot of nutrition hype around sweet potatoes, and rightly so! They are rich in fiber, potassium, vitamin C, vitamin B_5, and get their orange color from beta-carotene.

4 medium sweet potatoes, scrubbed and cut into ¼-inch slices

1 teaspoon sesame oil

2 tablespoons extra-virgin olive oil

3 teaspoons smoked paprika

3 teaspoons sesame seeds

Salt

Freshly ground black pepper

1. Preheat the oven to 425° F. Line a rimmed baking sheet with parchment paper.

2. Spread the sweet potato slices on the baking sheet and toss with sesame oil, olive oil, paprika, sesame seeds, and a pinch of salt and pepper.

3. Roast until tender and slightly browned, 20 to 25 minutes.

VARIATION: Add protein, such as chicken or salmon, to the same baking dish. Season the protein with the same ingredients and be sure to increase the cooking time 5 to 10 minutes to ensure that the meat is thoroughly cooked.

Per Serving Calories: 199; Fat: 10g; Saturated Fat: 1g; Sodium: 111mg; Cholesterol: 0mg; Carbs: 28g; Fiber: 5g; Sugar: 6g; Protein: 3g

Sweet Potatoes Stuffed with Swiss Chard

SERVES 4 / PREP TIME: 10 MINUTES / COOK TIME: 20 MINUTES

Swiss chard comes in many different shades, and all have anti-inflammatory and antioxidant properties due to its high amounts of beneficial compounds such as polyphenols and beta-carotene. This is a dish that looks sophisticated but is actually very easy to prepare. Goat cheese pairs well with this dish. Place a few crumbles on top of the cooked Swiss chard to create a creamy, tangy flavor profile.

4 medium sweet potatoes

2 tablespoons extra-virgin olive oil

1 small white onion, finely diced

Salt

1 bunch Swiss chard, stemmed and finely chopped

4 cloves garlic, grated or minced

½ teaspoon red pepper flakes

⅓ cup cooking sherry, Marsala wine, or chicken stock

1. Pierce the sweet potato skins with a fork 5 or 6 times. Microwave on high for 5 to 10 minutes, or until they are easily pierced and soft. Cut each potato in half.

2. Pour the olive oil in a large saucepan over medium-high heat. When the oil is hot and shimmering, add the onion and a pinch of salt. Cook, stirring occasionally, until onions are soft and translucent, about 5 minutes.

3. Add the Swiss chard, garlic, a pinch of salt, the red pepper flakes, and the sherry. Cook down until the sherry is thickened and the Swiss chard is soft, 3 to 5 minutes.

4. Spoon a quarter of the Swiss chard mixture onto each potato half.

PREPARATION TIP: To stem the chard, slice each leaf down the middle and cut out the stem. Slice the leaves into strips about ½-inch thick, then cross cut the strips to make a dice. Run your knife through the pile a few times for a finer dice.

Per Serving Calories: 211; Fat: 7g; Saturated Fat: 1g; Sodium: 228mg; Cholesterol: 0mg; Carbs: 32g; Fiber: 5g; Sugar: 7g; Protein: 3g

Spiced Crispy Chickpeas

SERVES 4 / PREP TIME: 10 MINUTES / COOK TIME: 12 MINUTES

Chickpeas contain both protein and fiber, which, when combined, slow digestion and help you feel fuller for longer. Their high carbohydrate content makes them great for snacking, too, as a little handful of chickpeas goes a long way.

1 tablespoon extra-virgin olive oil

1 small white onion, finely diced

Salt

2 (15-ounce) cans low-sodium chickpeas, drained and rinsed

2 cloves garlic, grated or minced

½ teaspoon red pepper flakes

1 teaspoon ground turmeric

Zest of 1 lemon

1. Heat a large saucepan over medium-high heat and pour in the olive oil. When the oil is hot and shimmering, add the onion and a pinch of salt. Cook, stirring occasionally, until the onions are soft and translucent, about 5 minutes.

2. Add the chickpeas and cook until they begin to crisp, about 5 minutes. Add the garlic, red pepper flakes, turmeric, and lemon zest. Cook until the garlic is fragrant, about 1 minute.

VARIATION: Add any fresh herbs you have on hand, such as rosemary and thyme, to give this recipe a different flavor profile.

Per Serving Calories: 244; Fat: 7g; Saturated Fat: 1g; Sodium: 49mg; Cholesterol: 0mg; Carbs: 36g; Fiber: 10g; Sugar: 7g; Protein: 11g

Protein-Packed Chickpea Spaghetti

SERVES 4 / PREP TIME: 3 MINUTES / COOK TIME: 15 MINUTES

We all need our pasta fix, but compared to regular or even whole-wheat spaghetti, chickpea spaghetti contains much more protein and fiber. You'll find lentil pasta in stores as well. Add leftover cooked veggies such as asparagus, mushrooms, and/or zucchini to this dish for an even more filling and healthier variation.

1 (8-ounce) box uncooked chickpea spaghetti

1 (24-ounce) jar low-sodium marinara sauce

1. Bring a large pot of water to boil over high heat.
2. Add the chickpea pasta and cook 2 minutes less than the directions on the box.
3. Strain pasta and add it back to the hot pot. Add the marinara sauce and heat until sauce is warmed through and the spaghetti is fully cooked.

INGREDIENT TIP: When choosing jarred marinara sauce, read the ingredients list for wholesome ingredients. Check the nutrition label for low sodium, and be sure it is 10 percent or less of the daily value.

Per Serving Calories: 264; Fat: 2g; Saturated Fat: 1g; Sodium: 54mg; Cholesterol: 0mg; Carbs: 55g; Fiber: 8g; Sugar: 9g; Protein: 9g

Smashed Black Beans

SERVES 4 / PREP TIME: 12 MINUTES / COOK TIME: 15 MINUTES

This recipe is a great alternative to refried beans, which are typically high in sodium and saturated fat. Black beans offer many nutritional benefits, one of which is aiding digestion with their high fiber content. Add fresh cilantro and lime juice before serving for a pop of bright flavor.

1 tablespoon extra-virgin olive oil

1 small white onion, finely diced

Salt

2 cloves garlic, grated or minced

½ teaspoon red pepper flakes

1 teaspoon smoked paprika

2 (15-ounce) cans low-sodium black beans, drained and rinsed

½ cup water

1. Heat a large saucepan over medium-high heat and pour in the olive oil. When it is hot and shimmering, add the onion and a pinch of salt. Cook, stirring occasionally, until the onions are soft and translucent, about 5 minutes.

2. Add the garlic, red pepper flakes, and smoked paprika. Cook for an additional minute, until all the spices are fragrant. Pour in the drained beans and water, stir to combine, cover, and cook for 5 minutes.

3. Reduce the heat to low and remove the lid. Use a potato masher or the back of a spoon to mash about half of the beans, or until your desired consistency. Continue to cook the beans uncovered, stirring often, about 3 minutes. If the beans seem dry, add a very small amount of water and stir to combine.

Per Serving Calories: 194; Fat: 4g; Saturated Fat: 1g; Sodium: 253mg; Cholesterol: 0mg; Carbs: 29g; Fiber: 13g; Sugar: 4g; Protein: 12g

Grilled Avocado Stuffed with Lentil Salad

SERVES 4 / PREP TIME: 12 MINUTES / COOK TIME: 3 MINUTES

Avocados are a good source of healthy fat. Fats aid in the absorption of fat-soluble vitamins, such as A, D, E, and K. Choose ripe but still firm avocados for this dish, and leave them in their jackets for grilling. Bruschetta is small grilled or toasted bread slices rubbed with garlic and topped with roasted peppers or tomatoes, olive oil, and salt. You can buy the pepper or tomato topping in jars in the grocery store.

1 (15-ounce) can black lentils, drained and rinsed

1 cup spinach, finely chopped

½ cup store-bought bruschetta spread

4 medium avocados, cut in half and seed removed

1 teaspoon extra-virgin olive oil

Salt

Freshly ground black pepper

1. Preheat a stovetop grill pan or a grill over medium heat.

2. In a medium bowl or storage container, mix the lentils, spinach, and bruschetta, and gently toss together.

3. Using the tip of a paring knife, score the flesh side of each avocado half in a crosshatch pattern. Brush the inside of the avocado halves with olive oil and sprinkle with salt and pepper.

4. Place the avocado halves cut-side down on the grill or grill pan for 2 to 3 minutes, until there are grill marks. Remove from grill pan and fill each half with the lentil mixture.

COST HACK: For the stuffing, use leftovers from the Lentil Bruschetta with Endive Scoops (page 143).

Per Serving Calories: 417; Fat: 30g; Saturated Fat: 4g; Sodium: 180mg; Cholesterol: 0mg; Carbs: 32g; Fiber: 19g; Sugar: 3g; Protein: 11g

Lime Quinoa

SERVES 4 / PREP TIME: 7 MINUTES / COOK TIME: 20 MINUTES

Here's a little-known fact about quinoa: It is actually a seed. Quinoa is very nutritionally dense and, unlike most grains, contains all nine essential amino acids, making it a great protein choice for vegetarians and vegans.

1 cup uncooked quinoa, rinsed

2 cups water

Zest and juice of 1 lime

Salt

Freshly ground black pepper

1. In a medium pot, pour in the quinoa and water. Bring to a boil over medium-high heat.

2. When it boils, reduce the heat to low, cover, and simmer until all the liquid is absorbed, 15 to 20 minutes.

3. Remove from heat and stir in the lime zest and juice, and a pinch of salt and pepper.

VARIATION: Using low-sodium chicken or vegetable stock instead of water gives this recipe a richer flavor. Omit the salt if you're using stock.

Per Serving Calories: 159; Fat: 3g; Saturated Fat: 0g; Sodium: 41mg; Cholesterol: 0mg; Carbs: 28g; Fiber: 3g; Sugar: 0g; Protein: 6g

Coconut Brown Rice

SERVES 4 / PREP TIME: 5 MINUTES / COOK TIME: 40 MINUTES

Coconut milk gives this rice a unique and slightly sweet taste. Brown rice contains roughly four times more fiber than white rice. Brown rice also contains higher amounts of antioxidants, vitamins, and minerals. Use brown jasmine rice, basmati, or short grain brown rice for this dish.

1 cup uncooked brown rice

1 cup light coconut milk

1¼ cups water

1-inch piece fresh ginger, peeled and sliced

Salt

1. In a medium pot, mix the rice, coconut milk, water, ginger, and a pinch of salt. Bring to a boil over medium heat.
2. When it boils, reduce the heat to low, cover, and simmer until all the liquid evaporates, 35 to 40 minutes. Remove from heat and fluff with a fork.

VARIATION: Add some unsweetened shredded coconut to the cooked rice to enhance the coconut flavor and give a nice texture to this recipe.

Per Serving Calories: 310; Fat: 16g; Saturated Fat: 13g; Sodium: 50mg; Cholesterol: 0mg; Carbs: 40g; Fiber: 3g; Sugar: 2g; Protein: 5g

Spanakopita Rice

SERVES 4 / PREP TIME: 10 MINUTES / COOK TIME: 45 MINUTES

Spanakopita is a savory Greek pie made of phyllo dough filled with spinach. In this dish, you get all the classic flavors of a crispy spanakopita in one healthy rice dish! This recipe uses fiber-rich spinach and brown rice, and also features a healthy amount of dill, which has antimicrobial and antioxidant properties.

1 tablespoon extra-virgin olive oil

½ small white onion, finely diced

2 cloves garlic, finely diced

1 cup uncooked brown rice

4 cups fresh spinach

2 cups low-sodium vegetable broth

¼ cup finely chopped fresh dill

Juice of ½ lemon

1. Heat large pot on medium-high heat and pour in the oil. Sauté the onion and garlic until the onions are translucent, about 5 minutes. Add the brown rice and spinach, and cook 1 to 2 minutes until the spinach is cooked down and the rice is slightly browned.

2. Add the broth and bring to a boil. Lower the heat, cover, and cook until rice is tender, 30 to 35 minutes.

3. When the rice is cooked, stir the pot to break up the spinach. Mix in the fresh dill and lemon juice just before serving.

COST HACK: You should have fresh dill left over from the Beet and Goat Cheese Frittata (page 68) or the Salmon Cakes (page 84), so plan to cook all three the same week.

Per Serving Calories: 231; Fat: 5g; Saturated Fat: 1g; Sodium: 69mg; Cholesterol: 0mg; Carbs: 41g; Fiber: 3g; Sugar: 1g; Protein: 6g

Mediterranean Farro Salad

SERVES 4 / PREP TIME: 12 MINUTES / COOK TIME: 35 MINUTES

Farro is a kind of whole-grain wheat that is loved for its toasted, nutty flavor. It's high in B vitamins and a contains a variety of minerals. With the arugula and fennel, this dish has a clean and fresh flavor, and features a light homemade vinaigrette you can use on any salad.

For the vinaigrette

3 tablespoons avocado oil

2 tablespoons red wine vinegar

¼ cup olive tapenade

1 teaspoon honey

Salt

Freshly ground black pepper

For the farro salad

1 cup uncooked farro, rinsed

3 cups water

Salt

1 large English cucumber, finely diced

2 cups chopped arugula

1 fennel bulb, finely chopped

1. To make the vinaigrette, in a medium bowl, whisk together the avocado oil, red wine vinegar, olive tapenade, honey, salt, and pepper until they are well combined. Set aside for the flavors to blend.

2. Put the farro, water, and a pinch of salt in a medium pot. Bring to a boil over medium-high heat, then reduce the heat to a simmer, cooking until the grains are al dente, 25 to 30 minutes. Remove from the heat and drain off any water that has not been absorbed.

3. Transfer the farro to a large mixing bowl or storage container, along with 2 cups of ice to cool it down. When ice has melted, drain the excess water and add the cucumber, arugula, and fennel, then combine. Pour on the vinaigrette and toss to coat.

STORAGE TIP: Serve immediately or cover and refrigerate for up to 2 days. This dish becomes more flavorful the longer it sits.

Per Serving Calories: 303; Fat: 16g; Saturated Fat: 2g; Sodium: 313mg; Cholesterol: 0mg; Carbs: 33g; Fiber: 7g; Sugar: 3g; Protein: 6g

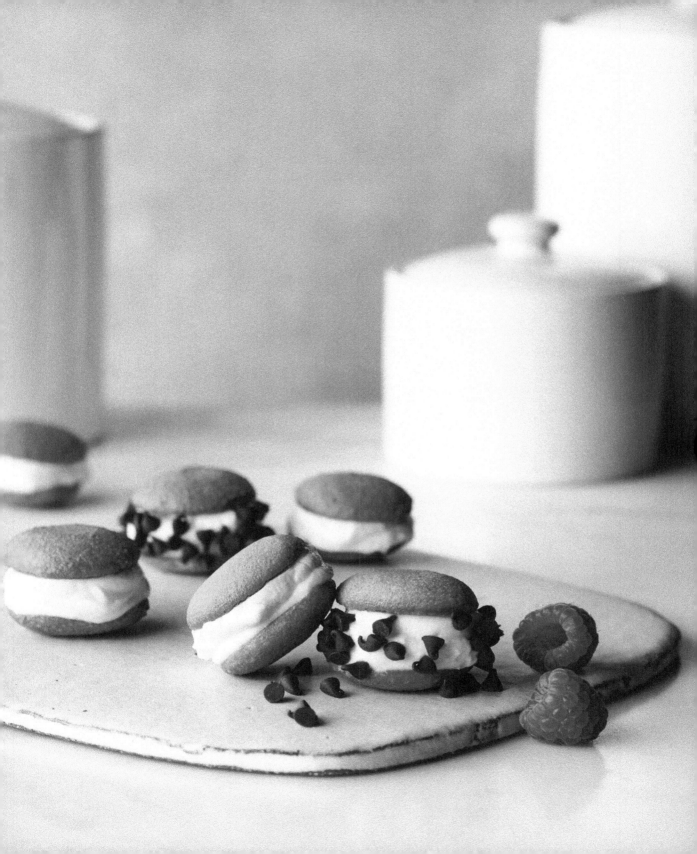

CHAPTER 7

Snacks and Sweets

Parmesan Popcorn with Pepitas

SERVES 2 / PREP TIME: 10 MINUTES

Parmesan, popcorn, and pepitas: perfection! Air-popped popcorn is a superb low-calorie snack that contains about 3.5 grams of fiber per 1-ounce serving. The addition of protein-filled pepitas (hulless pumpkin seeds) makes this a more substantial snack, keeping you fuller for longer. You can spray the popcorn for 3 to 5 seconds with olive oil cooking spray to add a healthy fat that will help the Parmesan stick better to the popcorn. You can also drizzle on 1 tablespoon or less of grass-fed butter, but remember that butter has saturated fat.

4 cups air-popped popcorn

½ cup pepitas

¼ cup grated Parmesan cheese

1. In a large bowl, combine popcorn, pepitas, and Parmesan cheese and toss gently to mix.

2. Portion into two containers, so you're not temped to eat the whole bowl!

COST HACK: Don't have an air popper? Just put some plain popcorn in a small brown paper bag, fold over the end, and put it in the microwave. Press the popcorn button and you will end up with perfectly popped popcorn without the expense and additives of microwave popcorn.

Per Serving Calories: 268; Fat: 18g; Saturated Fat: 5g; Sodium: 137mg; Cholesterol: 10mg; Carbs: 18g; Fiber: 3g; Sugar: 0g; Protein: 14g

Salty Sweet Trail Mix

SERVES 4 / PREP TIME: 5 MINUTES

The name says it all. We put a balanced spin on this trail mix with the addition of protein-filled pepitas and carbohydrates in Corn Chex. And, of course, chocolate—a necessary component in any trail mix—is provided with the addition of semi-sweet chocolate chips.

¼ cup Corn Chex cereal

¼ cup pepitas

¼ cup roasted almonds

¼ cup raw cashews

2 tablespoons semi-sweet chocolate chips

1. In a medium bowl or storage container, combine Corn Chex, pepitas, almonds, cashews, and chocolate chips and toss gently to mix.
2. Store in an airtight container for up to 7 days.

VARIATION: Substitute Wheat Chex or even popcorn for the Corn Chex. If you go with popcorn, increase the amount to 2 cups, since popcorn has fewer carbohydrate calories than Chex cereal.

Per Serving Calories: 171; Fat: 12g; Saturated Fat: 3g; Sodium: 17mg; Cholesterol: 0mg; Carbs: 12g; Fiber: 1g; Sugar: 5g; Protein: 5g

Chimichurri Hummus Cups with Carrots

SERVES 4 / PREP TIME: 5 MINUTES

Everyone knows about dipping carrots in hummus, so we decided to spice things up by tossing a zesty chimichurri into the mix. This is one of the quickest snacks in the book, and does one of the best jobs of holding hunger at bay due to the high fiber content in carrots and protein in hummus.

1 cup store-bought hummus

2 teaspoons store-bought chimichurri sauce

2 cups baby carrots

1. Place ¼ cup of hummus in 4 individual storage containers. Top each with ½ teaspoon chimichurri.

2. Serve with ½ cup or more of baby carrots.

PREPARATION TIP: Most grocery stores carry individual prepackaged baby carrots and hummus cups. Simply put ½ teaspoon of chimichurri in a small snack size zip-top bag to flavor the hummus, for an easy grab-and-go snack.

Per Serving Calories: 139; Fat: 7g; Saturated Fat: 1g; Sodium: 295mg; Cholesterol: 1mg; Carbs: 15g; Fiber: 5g; Sugar: 3g; Protein: 6g

Lentil Bruschetta with Endive Scoops

SERVES 4 / PREP TIME: 10 MINUTES

This is a super sophisticated-looking snack that is actually super simple and loaded with nutrients. Buying a fresh bruschetta spread from the refrigerated section of the store saves on time and number of ingredients, allowing you to whip this well-rounded snack together within minutes.

½ cup store-bought tomato or roasted pepper bruschetta spread

1 (15-ounce) can black lentils, drained and rinsed

1 cup finely chopped spinach

2 tablespoons crumbled feta cheese

12 endive leaves (about 2 heads)

1. In a large bowl, gently toss together the spread, lentils, spinach, and feta cheese.
2. Serve with endive leaves for dipping.

VARIATION: Exchange the endive leaves for celery sticks, or eat this salad in a lettuce cup or just with a fork. The feta can be swapped for 2 tablespoons of shredded Parmesan cheese or even 2 tablespoons of olive tapenade.

Per Serving Calories: 152; Fat: 4g; Saturated Fat: 1g; Sodium: 208mg; Cholesterol: 4mg; Carbs: 22g; Fiber: 11g; Sugar: 3g; Protein: 10g

Hemp Hearts and Chia-Crusted Avocado with Whole-Grain Crackers

SERVES 4 / PREP TIME: 7 MINUTES

This snack does especially well at keeping you full for a long time due to the high fat content in avocado and the high protein content in hemp and chia seeds. To top it all off, there's fiber and carbohydrates from the whole-wheat crackers.

2 large avocados

2 tablespoons hulled hemp seeds

1 tablespoon chia seeds

Lemon pepper

10 to 12 whole-wheat crackers

1. Slice the avocados in half, remove the pits, and cut each half into 3 wedges. Grasp the outer dark layer of skin and pull it away from the inner green flesh of the fruit. You can use a spoon to remove the flesh from the skin as well.

2. Sprinkle the avocado wedges with the hemp seeds, chia seeds, and pinch of lemon pepper.

3. Serve with whole-wheat crackers for dipping or spreading.

VARIATION: Exchange whole-wheat crackers for half a whole-wheat pita bread or a slice of toasted sourdough bread.

Per Serving Calories: 251; Fat: 19g; Saturated Fat: 3g; Sodium: 73mg; Cholesterol: 0mg; Carbs: 17g; Fiber: 9g; Sugar: 0g; Protein: 6g

Tzatziki Yogurt Sauce with Whole-Wheat Pita

SERVES 4 / PREP TIME: 10 MINUTES, PLUS 20 MINUTES TO BLEND

This snack holds you over from one meal to the next thanks to the protein and fat in Greek yogurt and the fiber in the whole-wheat pita. Tzatziki sauce itself is amazingly refreshing and is a versatile dipping sauce you can use for vegetables or other Mediterranean dishes. It is also a probiotic, meaning it contains beneficial bacteria, while whole-wheat pita is a prebiotic—a kind of dietary fiber that feeds healthy gut bacteria.

Juice of 1 lemon

2 tablespoons honey

Salt

Freshly ground black pepper

1 clove garlic, grated

4 tablespoons chopped fresh dill

1 to 2 tablespoons grated white onion

½ English cucumber, grated

1 (16-ounce) container plain 2-percent Greek yogurt

4 whole-wheat pitas

1. In a large bowl, combine the lemon juice, honey, and a pinch of salt and pepper. Stir until the honey and salt are dissolved.

2. Use a grater to finely shred the garlic into the lemon juice mixture. Then add the dill, onion, cucumber, and Greek yogurt and mix until they are well combined. Let rest 20 minutes for best flavor. Store up to a week in the refrigerator.

3. Serve with whole-wheat pita bread.

COST HACK: Pair any leftovers with Mediterranean Spiced Beef Meatballs (page 114) or Salmon Cakes (page 84). Use up the fresh dill in Spanakopita Rice (page 136).

Per Serving Calories: 294; Fat: 3g; Saturated Fat: 1g; Sodium: 434mg; Cholesterol: 10mg; Carbs: 51g; Fiber: 5g; Sugar: 14g; Protein: 18g

Marinated Cucumber and Tomato Salad

SERVES 4 / PREP TIME: 7 MINUTES, PLUS 15 MINUTES TO MARINATE

Cucumbers and tomatoes both contain high amounts of water and fiber, and together these keep you relatively full, making this an amazing and satisfying low-calorie snack. It's super fast and super simple, and it's smart to always have a little supply of this in the refrigerator. It will keep for about three days.

1 English cucumber, diced

1 pint cherry tomatoes, halved

3 tablespoons seasoned rice wine vinegar

¼ cup avocado oil

Red pepper flakes

1. In a large bowl, gently toss together English cucumber, cherry tomatoes, rice wine vinegar, avocado oil, and a pinch of red pepper flakes.

2. Let sit 10 to 15 minutes for the flavors to come together, then enjoy.

VARIATION: You can add radishes and red onions to this dish for more texture and flavor. This would also be great over a bed of lettuce, arugula, or mixed greens.

Per Serving Calories: 155; Fat: 14g; Saturated Fat: 2g; Sodium: 51mg; Cholesterol: 0mg; Carbs: 7g; Fiber: 2g; Sugar: 4g; Protein: 1g

Greek Watermelon Feta Salad

SERVES 4 / PREP TIME: 10 MINUTES

Watermelon and feta cheese might sound like an odd pairing, but we promise you'll be blown away by this salad! It's refreshing and different. Bring this dish to a backyard barbecue for a fun twist.

Juice of 1 lemon

2 tablespoons avocado oil

1 tablespoon olive tapenade

4 cups watermelon, cut in large cubes

¼ cup crumbled feta cheese

1. In a small bowl, whisk together the lemon juice, avocado oil, and olive tapenade to make the dressing.

2. In a large bowl, toss the dressing with the diced watermelon and feta.

VARIATION: You can use whole Kalamata olives instead of olive tapenade for a more chunky salad. Also try serving this over a bed of arugula for an added peppery flavor and even more texture.

Per Serving Calories: 143; Fat: 10g; Saturated Fat: 3g; Sodium: 159mg; Cholesterol: 8mg; Carbs: 12g; Fiber: 1g; Sugar: 10g; Protein: 2g

Cherry Tomato, Artichoke, and Mozzarella Skewers

SERVES 4 / PREP TIME: 10 MINUTES

The cherry (tomato) on top of this snack is the amazing nutritional profile of artichoke hearts. Artichokes aid in both digestion and liver health, and are completely loaded with fiber, containing around 7 grams of fiber per one medium artichoke heart.

20 cherry tomatoes

16 marinated mozzarella balls

16 marinated artichoke hearts

1. On 4 skewers, alternate cherry tomatoes, mozzarella balls, and artichoke hearts until each skewer has 5 cherry tomatoes, 4 mozzarella balls, and 4 artichoke hearts.

2. Serve immediately or store for up to 2 days in the refrigerator.

INGREDIENT TIP: Mozzarella balls are labeled according to their size. For this dish, choose *bocconcini* (Italian for bite-size) or *ciliegine* (Italian for cherry-size).

Per Serving Calories: 370; Fat: 28g; Saturated Fat: 16g; Sodium: 310mg; Cholesterol: 80mg; Carbs: 10g; Fiber: 5g; Sugar: 3g; Protein: 23g

Lime Chia Pudding

SERVES 2 / PREP TIME: 7 MINUTES, PLUS 30 MINUTES TO SET

When you mix chia seeds with any liquid and let them soak for a while, they absorb all the liquid's flavors and turn into a rich, delicious pudding—with no work at all! Chia seeds are superfoods that contain high amounts of omega-3 fatty acids, protein, fiber, and antioxidants, making this a wonderfully nutritious option for a dessert or snack.

1 cup light coconut milk, or any unsweetened nut milk

2 tablespoons chia seeds

Zest and juice of 1 lime

1 teaspoon honey

2 tablespoons slivered almonds

1. In a medium airtight container, mix coconut milk, chia seeds, lime zest and juice, and honey. Shake until well combined.

2. Let sit in the refrigerator 30 minutes or up to 24 hours for the pudding to set.

3. Top with slivered almonds just before serving.

VARIATION: Top this pudding with shredded unsweetened coconut, fresh berries, coconut whipped topping, or crushed whole-wheat graham crackers.

Per Serving Calories: 161; Fat: 10g; Saturated Fat: 1g; Sodium: 183mg; Cholesterol: 0mg; Carbs: 13g; Fiber: 7g; Sugar: 4g; Protein: 5g

Energizing Quinoa Parfait

SERVES 2 / PREP TIME: 10 MINUTES

This energizing quinoa parfait is not only filling, it is packed full of all the essential proteins your body needs to start the day or to recover from a workout. Quinoa is a powerhouse carbohydrate that is gluten-free, high in protein, high in fiber, and contains a variety of minerals needed to support metabolism.

1 cup cooked quinoa

1 cup plain 2-percent Greek yogurt

2 tablespoons slivered almonds

2 tablespoons unsalted pepitas

1 cup sliced fresh strawberries

Cinnamon, optional

1. Spoon ½ cup of cooked quinoa into the bottoms of two parfait glasses. Top each with ½ cup of yogurt, followed by 1 tablespoon of almonds, 1 tablespoon of pepitas, and ½ cup of sliced strawberries. Add a pinch of cinnamon on top, if using.
2. Serve immediately, or store in the refrigerator for 2 days.

COST HACK: You can use unsweetened frozen strawberries if fresh strawberries are not in season, or use any berries you have on hand. Mixed berries will bump up the antioxidants in this recipe.

Per Serving Calories: 386; Fat: 11g; Saturated Fat: 2g; Sodium: 66mg; Cholesterol: 10mg; Carbs: 49g; Fiber: 7g; Sugar: 9g; Protein: 23g

Frozen Yogurt Bark

SERVES 4 / PREP TIME: 7 MINUTES, PLUS 30 MINUTES TO FREEZE

What's fantastic about this yogurt bark is how easy and customizable it is. Substitute any topping, such as blueberries, unsweetened shredded coconut, nuts, or seeds. Keep a supply in your freezer and you'll always have something to snack on that is high in protein and will satisfy your sweet cravings.

2 cups low-fat vanilla Greek yogurt

½ cup fresh or frozen raspberries

1 tablespoon semi-sweet chocolate chips

2 tablespoons slivered almonds

1 tablespoon chia seeds

1. Line a rimmed baking sheet with wax paper or parchment paper.

2. Pour the Greek yogurt on the baking sheet and use a rubber spatula to smooth out until thin and even, about ¼- to ½-inch thick.

3. Sprinkle evenly with the raspberries, chocolate chips, almonds, and chia seeds and place in the freezer until firm, about 30 minutes. Break up into chucks and enjoy.

4. Store in the freezer, well wrapped, for up to 3 days.

Per Serving Calories: 147; Fat: 5g; Saturated Fat: 2g; Sodium: 66mg; Cholesterol: 5mg; Carbs: 21g; Fiber: 3g; Sugar: 7g; Protein: 6g

Raspberry Smash Frozen Yogurt Sandwich

SERVES 4 / PREP TIME: 10 MINUTES, PLUS 30 MINUTES TO FREEZE

This recipe is especially fun to assemble with friends or children for a cool afternoon snack or nighttime dessert. These miniature cookie sandwiches will satisfy sweet cravings while still providing protein from low-fat vanilla Greek yogurt and vitamin C from raspberries.

12 low-fat vanilla wafers

1 cup low-fat vanilla Greek yogurt

6 fresh or frozen raspberries

1. Line a shallow storage container with wax paper or parchment paper.

2. Lay out 6 wafers in the container. Put a small scoop of Greek yogurt (about 2 teaspoons) on each cookie. Put a raspberry in the middle of the yogurt. Top with another cookie, and press down lightly.

3. Place the container in the freezer for 25 to 30 minutes.

VARIATION: You can place a few mini chocolate chips around the raspberry for a chocolaty crunch.

Per Serving Calories: 137; Fat: 3g; Saturated Fat: 1g; Sodium: 89mg; Cholesterol: 12mg; Carbs: 4g; Fiber: 2g; Sugar: 15g; Protein: 24g

Coconut Whip with Mixed Berries

SERVES 2 / PREP TIME: 2 MINUTES / COOK TIME: 1 MINUTE

Berries and cream is a classic combination. Using a coconut whipped topping (such as CocoWhip) rather than a dairy whip offers more healthy fats that will help you stay full after enjoying this relatively light but seriously delicious dessert.

1 cup unsweetened frozen mixed berries, thawed

¼ cup store-bought coconut whipped topping

1 teaspoon chia seeds

2 tablespoons slivered almonds

Unsweetened cocoa powder, optional

1. Place ½ cup frozen berries in the bottom of 2 microwave-safe bowls. Microwave 1 minute on high.

2. Top each bowl with 2 tablespoons of coconut whip, ½ teaspoon of chia seeds, and 1 tablespoon of slivered almonds.

3. Add a pinch of unsweetened cocoa powder on top of each serving, if using.

VARIATION: Use any frozen fruit you have on hand. Try adding a few chocolate chips on top.

Per Serving Calories: 147; Fat: 8g; Saturated Fat: 3g; Sodium: 0mg; Cholesterol: 1mg; Carbs: 21g; Fiber: 3g; Sugar: 12g; Protein: 2g

Three-Minute Berry Crumble

SERVES 2 / PREP TIME: 5 MINUTES / COOK TIME: 3 MINUTES

What tops off your day better than a fresh berry crumble? Berries are loaded with antioxidants and provide the natural sugars you need to satisfy any sweet cravings. In addition, this recipe uses frozen berries, which cut down on both cost and prep time.

1 cup unsweetened frozen mixed berries

1 cup uncooked rolled oats

1 teaspoon chia seeds

1 teaspoon cinnamon

2 teaspoons brown sugar

1 tablespoon grass-fed butter or coconut oil

Salt

1. Place ½ cup frozen berries in the bottoms of two microwave-safe bowls.

2. In a small bowl, combine the rolled oats, chia seeds, cinnamon, brown sugar, butter, and a pinch of salt. Spoon half the crumble mixture over the frozen berries in each bowl.

3. Microwave on high for 3 minutes, until the berries are hot and the crumble is softened.

VARIATION: You can use fresh diced apples rather than berries here. Use 1 apple for 2 servings and leave the skin on the apple; it has lots of healthy fiber.

Per Serving Calories: 276; Fat: 10g; Saturated Fat: 0g; Sodium: 81mg; Cholesterol: 0mg; Carbs: 42g; Fiber: 7g; Sugar: 11g; Protein: 6g

Protein-Packed Cottage Cheese Bowl with Berries

SERVES 2 / PREP TIME: 5 MINUTES

Cottage cheese is the perfect creamy, protein-packed indulgence. All that protein content makes this a filling snack that will also keep your metabolism stable throughout the day. The berries not only add sweet flavor, but also have fiber that keeps you satisfied until the next meal. Use organic fresh berries if you prefer.

1 cup low-fat cottage cheese

1 cup unsweetened frozen mixed berries, thawed

1 teaspoon chia seeds

Cinnamon, optional

1. Place ½ cup of the cottage cheese in the bottoms of two bowls. Top each with ½ cup thawed berries and ½ teaspoon chia seeds.

2. Add a pinch of cinnamon on top of each serving, if using.

3. Serve immediately or store in the refrigerator for 2 days.

STORAGE TIP: Make these in glass jars that you can grab on the go for a quick and easy snack.

Per Serving Calories: 144; Fat: 3g; Saturated Fat: 2g; Sodium: 380mg; Cholesterol: 9mg; Carbs: 12g; Fiber: 5g; Sugar: 4g; Protein: 17g

Pillowy Lemon Ricotta with Macerated Strawberries

SERVES 2 / PREP TIME: 10 MINUTES, PLUS 15 MINUTES TO MARINATE

We love adding fruit to any dessert for natural sweetness. Notice this recipe only uses 2 teaspoons of honey. But feel free to omit it entirely if your berries are extra ripe.

1 cup low-fat ricotta cheese

Zest and juice of 1 lemon

2 teaspoons honey, divided

1 teaspoon pure vanilla extract

Salt

½ pound strawberries, hulled and chopped

1. In a medium bowl, add the ricotta, lemon zest, 1 teaspoon of honey, vanilla extract, and a pinch of salt. Mix until the ricotta is whipped and pillowy. Set aside.

2. In a large bowl, toss the chopped strawberries with the lemon juice and 1 teaspoon honey. Mash slightly with a fork. Let sit 10 to 15 minutes.

3. Divide the ricotta mixture between two bowls and top each with half the macerated strawberries.

PREPARATION TIP: You can prepare the strawberries in step 2 before you start cooking dinner and set them aside to sit and macerate while you cook. You can also assemble the whole thing and keep the bowls covered in the refrigerator for up to 4 hours.

Per Serving Calories: 78; Fat: 3g; Saturated Fat: 2g; Sodium: 81mg; Cholesterol: 10mg; Carbs: 9g; Fiber: 1g; Sugar: 6g; Protein: 4g

Baked Peaches Topped with Matcha Granola

SERVES 4 / PREP TIME: 10 MINUTES / COOK TIME: 20 MINUTES

If you've never cooked with matcha, you'll love the delicious flavor it can add to any dessert. Matcha does contain caffeine, so be sure to limit how much you use. Toss in any nuts and seeds you have on hand. And for extra decadence, top each peach with 2 tablespoons of store-bought coconut whip.

2 peaches, halved and pitted

2 cups uncooked rolled oats

1 tablespoon matcha green tea powder

½ cup slivered almonds

½ cup pepitas

¼ teaspoon salt

¼ cup coconut oil, melted

⅓ cup honey

1 tablespoon pure vanilla extract

1. Preheat the oven to 325° F. Line 2 rimmed baking sheets with parchment paper.

2. On one baking sheet, place the peaches cut side down.

3. In a large mixing bowl, add the rolled oats, matcha powder, almonds, pepitas, salt, coconut oil, honey, and vanilla extract. Gently stir to combine and make sure everything is well coated. Use a rubber spatula to spread this mixture in an even layer on the other baking sheet.

4. Place both baking sheets in the oven and bake for 10 minutes. Toss the granola and bake for another 5 to 10 minutes, until the granola is slightly browned and fragrant. Keep a close eye on it during the last 5 minutes so it doesn't burn.

5. Take both baking sheets out of the oven and assemble hot or cooled. Place 3 heaping tablespoons of matcha granola on each baked peach half to serve.

STORAGE TIP: You can make this healthy granola and store it in an airtight container for up to 1 week. This granola would be great over yogurt in the morning or on top of some frozen fruit with coconut whip for dessert.

Per Serving Calories: 569; Fat: 32g; Saturated Fat: 15g; Sodium: 154mg; Cholesterol: 0mg; Carbs: 64g; Fiber: 7g; Sugar: 32g; Protein: 14g

Crunchy Chocolate Peanut Butter Cups

SERVES 4 / PREP TIME: 15 MINUTES, PLUS 10 MINUTES TO CHILL / COOK TIME: 2 MINUTES

Who can deny themselves a chocolate peanut butter cup of goodness? You may be surprised to know that these little morsels are actually high in both protein and fiber, thanks to the addition of hemp seeds and puffed brown rice. Puffed brown rice, also called brown rice crisps, is like Rice Krispies, only healthier. You can find it in many supermarkets and most health food stores.

½ cup peanut butter

¼ cup hulled hemp seeds

¼ cup puffed brown rice

Salt

½ cup semi-sweet chocolate chips

1 teaspoon coconut oil

Nonstick cooking spray

1. In a small microwave-safe bowl, microwave the peanut butter until melted, about 1 minute. Stir in the hemp seeds, puffed brown rice, and a pinch of salt.

2. In a separate small microwave-safe bowl, combine the chocolate chips and coconut oil. Microwave 1 minute on high until the chocolate is melted.

3. Line an 8-cup muffin tin with paper liners and spray them inside with nonstick cooking spray. Put 1 heaping tablespoon of the peanut butter mixture in the bottom of each cup and top with 1 tablespoon of the melted chocolate mixture.

4. Pop in the freezer for 10 minutes to harden.

VARIATION: You can also make this into bars. Line a medium food storage container with parchment paper and spread the peanut butter mixture in the container. Top with the chocolate mixture. Let cool and cut into 8 bars.

Per Serving Calories: 422; Fat: 29g; Saturated Fat: 10g; Sodium: 187mg; Cholesterol: 0mg; Carbs: 29g; Fiber: 3g; Sugar: 19g; Protein: 13g

Stovetop Chocolate Zucchini Oat Pudding

SERVES 2 / PREP TIME: 10 MINUTES / COOK TIME: 15 MINUTES

This is a great recipe for getting your chocolate fix while still packing a nutritional punch. The water-soluble fiber in oats has a gel-like property that forms a natural pudding texture. The zucchini bits will blend away into the mix and you'll have no idea that a vegetable is hidden in this delicious chocolate pudding. Top this with coconut whip, mini chocolate chips, or banana slices.

1 cup water

⅓ cup uncooked rolled oats

1 tablespoon ground flaxseed

1 tablespoon unsweetened cocoa powder

Cinnamon

Salt

½ banana, sliced

½ cup finely grated zucchini

¼ cup egg whites

½ teaspoon pure vanilla extract

1. In a medium pot, bring the water to a boil. Add the oats, ground flaxseed, cocoa powder, a pinch of cinnamon and salt, and reduce the heat. Cook 2 minutes, then add the banana and zucchini. Stir frequently to break up the fruit and veggies. Cook on medium-low heat until the liquid is absorbed, about 5 minutes.

2. Add the egg whites and stir vigorously for 2 minutes, until the oats are fluffy and the egg whites are incorporated. Then add the vanilla extract.

3. Turn off the heat, cover, and let sit for 5 minutes before serving.

Per Serving Calories: 100; Fat: 2g; Saturated Fat: 1g; Sodium: 113mg; Cholesterol: 0mg; Carbs: 15g; Fiber: 4g; Sugar: 5g; Protein: 6g

MONDAY

BREAKFAST

LUNCH

DINNER

SNACK 1

SNACK 2

TUESDAY

BREAKFAST

LUNCH

DINNER

SNACK 1

SNACK 2

WEDNESDAY

BREAKFAST

LUNCH

DINNER

SNACK 1

SNACK 2

THURSDAY

BREAKFAST

LUNCH

DINNER

SNACK 1

SNACK 2

FRIDAY

BREAKFAST

LUNCH

DINNER

SNACK 1

SNACK 2

SATURDAY

BREAKFAST

LUNCH

DINNER

SNACK 1

SNACK 2

SUNDAY

BREAKFAST

LUNCH

DINNER

SNACK 1

SNACK 2

THE DIRTY DOZEN™ AND THE CLEAN FIFTEEN™

A nonprofit environmental watchdog organization called Environmental Working Group (EWG) looks at data supplied by the US Department of Agriculture (USDA) and the Food and Drug Administration (FDA) about pesticide residues. Each year it compiles a list of the best and worst pesticide loads found in commercial crops. You can use these lists to decide which fruits and vegetables to buy organic to minimize your exposure to pesticides and which produce is considered safe enough to buy conventionally. This does not mean they are pesticide-free, though, so wash these fruits and vegetables thoroughly. The list is updated annually, and you can find it online at EWG.org/FoodNews.

Dirty Dozen™

1. strawberries
2. spinach
3. kale
4. nectarines
5. apples
6. grapes
7. peaches
8. cherries
9. pears
10. tomatoes
11. celery
12. potatoes

Additionally, nearly three-quarters of hot pepper samples contained pesticide residues.

Clean Fifteen™

1. avocados
2. sweet corn
3. pineapples
4. sweet peas (frozen)
5. onions
6. papayas
7. eggplants
8. asparagus
9. kiwis
10. cabbages
11. cauliflower
12. cantaloupes
13. broccoli
14. mushrooms
15. honeydew melons

MEASUREMENT CONVERSIONS

Volume Equivalents (Liquid)

US Standard	US Standard (ounces)	Metric (approximate)
2 tablespoons	1 fl. oz.	30 mL
¼ cup	2 fl. oz.	60 mL
½ cup	4 fl. oz.	120 mL
1 cup	8 fl. oz.	240 mL
1½ cups	12 fl. oz.	355 mL
2 cups or 1 pint	16 fl. oz.	475 mL
4 cups or 1 quart	32 fl. oz.	1 L
1 gallon	128 fl. oz.	4 L

Oven Temperatures

Fahrenheit	Celsius (approximate)
250°F	120°C
300°F	150°C
325°F	165°C
350°F	180°C
375°F	190°C
400°F	200°C
425°F	220°C
450°F	230°C

Volume Equivalents (Dry)

US Standard	Metric (approximate)
⅛ teaspoon	0.5mL
¼ teaspoon	1mL
½ teaspoon	2mL
¾ teaspoon	4mL
1 teaspoon	5mL
1 tablespoon	15mL
¼ cup	59mL

Weight Equivalents

US Standard	Metric (approximate)
½ ounce	15g
1 ounce	30g
2 ounces	60g
4 ounces	115g
8 ounces	225g
12 ounces	340g
16 ounces or 1 pound	455g

REFERENCES

Chapter One

"Basic Report: 01123, Egg, Whole, Raw, Fresh." USDA Food Composition Databases. April 2018. https://ndb.nal.usda.gov/ndb/foods/show/112.

"Basic Report: 12006, Seeds, Chia Seeds, Dried." USDA Food Composition Databases. April 2018. https://ndb.nal.usda.gov/ndb/foods/show/12006.

Bowling, Nicole. "Cruciferous Vegetables: Health Benefits and Recipes." *Healthline*. October 11, 2017. https://www.healthline.com/health/food-nutrition/crucifeous-vegetables#1.

Burgess, Lana. "What Are the Benefits of Milk Thistle?" Medical News Today. Accessed August 29, 2019. https://www.medicalnewstoday.com/articles/320362.php.

Chainani-Wu, Nita. "Safety and Anti-Inflammatory Activity of Curcumin: A Component of Tumeric (*Curcuma Longa*)." *The Journal of Alternative and Complementary Medicine* 9, no. 1 (July 5, 2004): 161–68. https://doi.org/10.1089/107555303321223035.

Coutinho, Diego De Sá, Maria Pacheco, Rudimar Frozza, and Andressa Bernardi. "Anti-Inflammatory Effects of Resveratrol: Mechanistic Insights." *International Journal of Molecular Sciences* 19, no. 6 (2018): 1812. https://doi.org/10.3390/ijms19061812.

González-Périz, Ana, et al. "Obesity-Induced Insulin Resistance and Hepatic Steatosis Are Alleviated by ω-3 Fatty Acids: A Role for Resolvins and Protectins." *The FASEB Journal* 23, no. 6 (June 2009): 1946–57. https://doi.org/10.1096/fj.08-125674.

Goodson, Amy. "Why Turmeric and Black Pepper Is a Powerful Combination." *Healthline*. July 4, 2018. https://www.healthline.com/nutrition/turmeric-and-black-pepper#active-ingredients.

Gunnars, Kris. "Fruit Juice Is Just as Unhealthy as a Sugary Drink." *Healthline*. June 4, 2017. https://www.healthline.com/nutrition/fruit-juice-is-just-as-bad-as-soda#section3.

Gunnars, Kris. "Grass-Fed vs. Grain-Fed Beef—What's the Difference?" *Healthline*. May 7, 2018. htttps://www.healthline.com/nutrition/grass-fed-vs-grain-fed-beef.

Guo, Yu, Suli Wang, Ying Wang, and Tiehong Zhu. "Silymarin Improved Diet-Induced Liver Damage and Insulin Resistance by Decreasing Inflammation in Mice." *Pharmaceutical Biology* 54, no. 12 (December 8, 2016): 2995–3000. https://doi.org/10.1080/13880209.2016.1199042.

Gupta, Subash C., Sridevi Patchva, and Bharat B. Aggarwal. "Therapeutic Roles of Curcumin: Lessons Learned from Clinical Trials." *The AAPS Journal* 15, no. 1 (January 2013): 195–218. https://doi.org/10.1208/s12248-012-9432-8.

Holt, Susanne H. A., and Janette Brand Miller. "Increased Insulin Responses to Ingested Foods Are Associated with Lessened Satiety." *Appetite* 24, no. 1 (February 1995): 43–54. https://doi.org/10.1016/s0195-6663(95)80005-0.

Kim, Hyun Min, and Jaetaek Kim. "The Effects of Green Tea on Obesity and Type 2 Diabetes." *Diabetes & Metabolism Journal* 37, no. 3 (June 14, 2013): 173. https://doi.org/10.4093/dmj.2013.37.3.173.

Krajka-Kuźniak, Violetta, Jarosław Paluszczak, Hanna Szaefer, and Wanda Baer-Dubowska. "Betanin, a Beetroot Component, Induces Nuclear Factor Erythroid-2-Related Factor 2-Mediated Expression of Detoxifying/Antioxidant Enzymes in Human Liver Cell Lines." *British Journal of Nutrition* 110, no. 12 (December 28, 2013): 2138–49. https://doi.org/10.1017/s0007114513001645.

Javidi, Afrooz, Hassan Mozaffari-Khosravi, Azadeh Nadjarzadeh, Ali Dehghani, and Mohammadhassan Eftekhari. "The Effect of Flaxseed Powder on Insulin Resistance Indices and Blood Pressure in Prediabetic Individuals: A Randomized Controlled Clinical Trial." *Journal of Research in Medical Sciences* 21, no. 1 (September 1, 2016): 70. https://doi.org/10.4103/1735-1995.189660.

Overall, John, et al. "Metabolic Effects of Berries with Structurally Diverse Anthocyanins." *International Journal of Molecular Sciences* 18, no. 2 (February 15, 2017): 422. https://doi.org/10.3390/ijms18020422.

Peng, Xiaoli, et al. "Effect of Green Tea Consumption on Blood Pressure: A Meta-Analysis of 13 Randomized Controlled Trials." *Scientific Reports* 4, no. 1 (September 1, 2014). https://doi.org/10.1038/srep06251.

Shenker, Maura. "Foods That Are Good for a Liver Cleanse." Livestrong.com. Accessed August 29, 2019. https://www.livestrong.com/article /322704-foods-that-are-good-for-a-liver-cleanse/.

Surai, Peter. "Silymarin as a Natural Antioxidant: An Overview of the Current Evidence and Perspectives." *Antioxidants* 4, no. 1 (March 20, 2015): 204–47. https://doi.org/10.3390/antiox4010204.

Tinsley, Grant. "6 Benefits of Reishi Mushroom (Plus Side Effects and Dosage)." *Healthline*. March 31, 2018. https://www.healthline.com /nutrition/reishi-mushroom-benefits#section5.

Xiao, Chun, et al. "Hypoglycemic Effects of Ganoderma Lucidum Polysaccharides in Type 2 Diabetic Mice." *Archives of Pharmacal Research* 35, no. 10 (October 2012): 1793–1801. https://doi.org/10.1007/s12272-012-1012-z.

Zhu, Xiangyun, et al. "Effects of Resveratrol on Glucose Control and Insulin Sensitivity in Subjects with Type 2 Diabetes: Systematic Review and Meta-Analysis." *Nutrition & Metabolism* 14, no. 1 (September 22, 2017). https://doi.org/10.1186/s12986-017-0217-z.

Chapter Three

Asgary, Sedigheh, Shaghayeghhaghjoo Javanmard, and Aida Zarfeshany. "Potent Health Effects of Pomegranate." *Advanced Biomedical Research* 3, no. 1 (March 25, 2014): 100. https://doi.org/10.4103/ 2277-9175.129371.

"Basic Report: 15076, Fish, Salmon, Atlantic, Wild, Raw." USDA Food Composition Databases. April 2018. https://ndb.nal.usda.gov/ndb/foods /show/15076.

Bischoff-Ferrari, Heike. "Health Effects of Vitamin D." *Dermatologic Therapy* 23, no. 1 (2010): 23–30. https://doi.org/10.1111/j.1529-8019.2009.01288.x.

Ekanayaka, R. A. I., N. K. Ekanayaka, B. Perera, and P. G. S. M. De Silva. "Impact of a Traditional Dietary Supplement with Coconut Milk and Soya Milk on the Lipid Profile in Normal Free Living Subjects." *Journal of Nutrition and Metabolism* 2013 (October 24, 2013): 1–11. https://doi .org/10.1155/ 2013/ 481068.

"Full Report (All Nutrients): 45363296, ARTICHOKES, UPC: 000651702506." USDA Food Composition Databases. July 2018. https://ndb.nal.usda.gov /ndb/foods/show/45363296?.

Krajka-Kuźniak, Violetta, et al. "Betanin, a Beetroot Component, Induces Nuclear Factor Erythroid-2-Related Factor 2-Mediated Expression of Detoxifying/Antioxidant Enzymes in Human Liver Cell Lines." *British Journal of Nutrition* 110, no. 12 (December 17, 2013): 2138–49. https://doi.org/10.1017/s0007114513001645.

Nugent, A. P. "Health Properties of Resistant Starch." *Nutrition Bulletin* 30, no. 1 (February 16, 2005): 27–54. https://doi.org/10.1111/j.1467-3010.2005.00481.x.

Olas, Beata. "Berry Phenolic Antioxidants—Implications for Human Health?" *Frontiers in Pharmacology* 9 (March 26, 2018). https://doi.org/10.3389/fphar.2018.00078.

Rasane, Prasad, et al. "Nutritional Advantages of Oats and Opportunities for Its Processing as Value Added Foods—A Review." *Journal of Food Science and Technology* 52, no. 2 (February 25, 2013): 662–75. https://doi.org/10.1007/s13197-013-1072-1.

Rodriguez-Leyva, Delfin, et al. "The Cardiovascular Effects of Flaxseed and Its Omega-3 Fatty Acid, Alpha-Linolenic Acid." *Canadian Journal of Cardiology* 26, no. 9 (November 2010): 489–96. https://doi.org/10.1016/s0828-282x(10)70455-4.

Taga, M. Silvia, E. E. Miller, and D. E. Pratt. "Chia Seeds as a Source of Natural Lipid Antioxidants." *Journal of the American Oil Chemists' Society* 61, no. 5 (May 1984): 928–31. https://doi.org/10.1007/bf02542169.

Weiss, David J., and Christopher R. Anderton. "Determination of Catechins in Matcha Green Tea by Micellar Electrokinetic Chromatography." *Journal of Chromatography A* 1011, no. 1-2 (September 2003): 173–80. https://doi.org/10.1016/s0021-9673(03)01133-6.

Chapter Four

"Basic Report: 15015, Fish, Cod, Atlantic, Raw." USDA Food Composition Databases. April 2018. https://ndb.nal.usda.gov/ndb/foods/show/15015.

"Basic Report: 15102, Fish, Snapper, Mixed Species, Cooked, Dry Heat." USDA Food Composition Databases. April 2018. https://ndb.nal.usda.gov/ndb/foods/show/4584.

"Basic Report: 15127, Fish, Tuna, Fresh, Yellowfin, Raw." USDA Food Composition Databases. April 2018. https://ndb.nal.usda.gov/ndb/foods/show/15127.

"Citrus Peel Extract Shown to Reduce Insulin Resistance; May Help Diabetics, Says Research." *Natural News*, June 20, 2006. https://www.naturalnews.com/019430.html.

Costa, Anita. "Nutrition: The Health Benefits of Citrus Peels." *Best Health Magazine Canada*, January 19, 2018. https://www.besthealthmag.ca/best-eats/nutrition/nutrition-the-health-benefits-of-citrus-peels/.

"Full Report (All Nutrients): 45208935, TILAPIA FILLETS, UPC: 011150572293." USDA Food Composition Databases. July 2018. https://ndb.nal.usda.gov/ndb/foods/show/45208935.

Hodges, Romilly E., and Deanna M. Minich. "Modulation of Metabolic Detoxification Pathways Using Foods and Food-Derived Components: A Scientific Review with Clinical Application." *Journal of Nutrition and Metabolism* 2015 (June 16, 2015): 1–23. https://doi.org/10.1155/2015/760689.

Köhrle, Josef. "Selenium and the Control of Thyroid Hormone Metabolism." *Thyroid* 15, no. 8 (August 2005): 841–53. https://doi.org/10.1089/thy.2005.15.841.

Lucas, Grace. "Gut Thinking: The Gut Microbiome and Mental Health beyond the Head." *Microbial Ecology in Health and Disease* 29, no. 2 (November 30, 2018): 1548250. https://doi.org/10.1080/16512235.2018.1548250.

Nayar, N M., and K. L. Mehra. "Sesame: Its Uses, Botany, Cytogenetics, and Origin." *Economic Botany* 24, no. 1 (January 1970): 20–31. https://doi.org/10.1007/bf02860629.

Okada, Yoshikiyo, et al. "Tu2021 Anti-Inflammatory Effect of Novel Probiotic Yeasts Isolated from Japanese 'Miso' on DSS-Induced Colitis." *Gastroenterology* 150, no. 4 (April 2016). https://doi.org/10.1016/s0016-5085(16)33413-8.

Pirasath, S., K. Thayaananthan, S. Balakumar, and V. Arasaratnam. "Effect of Dietary Curries on the Glycaemic Index." *Ceylon Medical Journal* 55, no. 4 (December 29, 2010): 118. https://doi.org/10.4038/cmj.v55i4.2629.

Chapter Five

Akbari-Fakhrabadi, Maryam, Javad Heshmati, Mahdi Sepidarkish, and Farzad Shidfar. "Effect of Sumac (Rhus Coriaria) on Blood Lipids: A Systematic Review and Meta-Analysis." *Complementary Therapies in Medicine* 40 (October 2018): 8–12. https://doi.org/10.1016/j.ctim.2018.07.001.

Arnarson, Atli. "Chili Peppers 101: Nutrition Facts and Health Effects." *Healthline*. May 13, 2019. https://www.healthline.com/nutrition/foods/chili-peppers#vitamins-and-minerals.

"Basic Report: 02014, Spices, Cumin Seed." USDA Food Composition Databases. April 2018. https://ndb.nal.usda.gov/ndb/foods/show/02014.

"Basic Report: 02049, Thyme, Fresh." USDA Food Composition Databases. April 2018. https://ndb.nal.usda.gov/ndb/foods/show/02049.

"Basic Report: 11260, Mushrooms, White, Raw." USDA Food Composition Databases. April 2018. https://ndb.nal.usda.gov/ndb/foods/show/11260.

"Basic Report: 16112, Miso." USDA Food Composition Databases. April 2018. https://ndb.nal.usda.gov/ndb/foods/show/4849.

Bhandari, Prasanr. "Garlic (Allium Sativum L.): A Review of Potential Therapeutic Applications." *International Journal of Green Pharmacy* 6, no. 2 (2012): 118–29. https://www.greenpharmacy.info/index.php/ijgp/article/view/247.

Bodagh, Mehrnaz Nikkhah, Iradj Maleki, and Azita Hekmatdoost. "Ginger in Gastrointestinal Disorders: A Systematic Review of Clinical Trials." *Food Science & Nutrition* 7, no. 1 (November 5, 2018): 96–108. https://doi.org/10.1002/fsn3.807.

Chilla, C., D.A. Guillén, C.G. Barroso, and J.A. Pérez-Bustamante. "Automated on-Line-Solid-Phase Extraction—High-Performance Liquid Chromatography-Diode Array Detection of Phenolic Compounds in Sherry Wine." *Journal of Chromatography A* 750, no. 1–2 (October 25, 1996): 209–14. https://doi.org/10.1016/0021-9673(96)00557-2.

Descalzo, A. M., et al. "Antioxidant Status and Odour Profile in Fresh Beef from Pasture or Grain-Fed Cattle." *Meat Science* 75, no. 2 (February 2007): 299–307. https://doi.org/10.1016/j.meatsci.2006.07.015.

Dhaheri, Yusra Al, et al. "Anti-Metastatic and Anti-Tumor Growth Effects of Origanum Majorana on Highly Metastatic Human Breast Cancer Cells: Inhibition of NFκB Signaling and Reduction of Nitric Oxide

Production." *PLoS ONE* 8, no. 7 (July 10, 2013). https://doi.org/10.1371/journal.pone.0068808.

Mitchell, Peter. "Effects of Capsaicin on Digestion." Livestrong.com. Accessed September 10, 2019. https://www.livestrong.com/article/483294-effects-of-capsaicin-on-digestion/.

Egbuonu, Anthony, and Chigozirim Osuji. "Proximate Compositions and Antibacterial Activity of Citrus Sinensis (Sweet Orange) Peel and Seed Extracts." *European Journal of Medicinal Plants* 12, no. 3 (February 5, 2016): 1–7. https://doi.org/10.9734/ejmp/2016/24122.

Fanous, Summer. "Are Cashews Good for You?" *Healthline*. May 11, 2019. https://www.healthline.com/health/are-cashews-good-for-you.

"Full Report (All Nutrients): 02009, Spices, Chili Powder." USDA Food Composition Databases. April 2018. https://ndb.nal.usda.gov/ndb/foods/show/02009.

"Full Report (All Nutrients): 02031, Spices, Pepper, Red or Cayenne." USDA Food Composition Databases. April 2018. https://ndb.nal.usda.gov/ndb/foods/show/02031.

"Full Report (All Nutrients): 45338590, HATCH GREEN CHILE, UPC: 815800020024." USDA Food Composition Databases. July 2018. https://ndb.nal.usda.gov/ndb/foods/show/45338590.

Janssens, Pilou L. H. R., et al. "Acute Effects of Capsaicin on Energy Expenditure and Fat Oxidation in Negative Energy Balance." *PLoS ONE* 8, no. 7 (July 2, 2013). https://doi.org/10.1371/journal.pone.0067786.

Johri, RK. "Cuminum Cyminum and Carum Carvi: An Update." *Pharmacognosy Reviews* 5, no. 9 (2011): 63. https://doi.org/10.4103/0973-7847.79101.

Kemmerich, Bernd, Reinhild Eberhardt, and Holger Stammer. "Efficacy and Tolerability of a Fluid Extract Combination of Thyme Herb and Ivy Leaves and Matched Placebo in Adults Suffering from Acute Bronchitis with Productive Cough: A Prospective, Double-Blind, Placebo-Controlled Trial." *Arzneimittelforschung* 56, no. 09 (2006): 652–60. https://doi.org/10.1055/s-0031-1296767.

Ware, Megan, RDN LD. "What Is the Nutritional Value of Mushrooms?" Medical News Today. February 23, 2017. https://www.medicalnewstoday.com/articles/278858.php.

Leyva-Lopez, Nayely, et al. "Essential Oils of Oregano: Biological Activity beyond Their Antimicrobial Properties." *Molecules* 22, no. 6 (June 14, 2017): 989. https://doi.org/10.3390/molecules22060989.

Link, Rachael. "The Heart-Healthy, Bone-Supporting Antioxidant Herb." Dr. Axe, September 1, 2018. https://draxe.com/nutrition/herbs/sumac-spice/.

"Lutein & Zeaxanthin." American Optometric Association. Accessed September 10, 2019. https://www.aoa.org/patients-and-public/caring-for-your-vision/diet-and-nutrition/lutein.

Mcafee, A. J., et al. "Red Meat from Animals Offered a Grass Diet Increases Platelet n–3 PUFA in Healthy Consumers." *Proceedings of the Nutrition Society* 69, no. OCE4 (2010). https://doi.org/10.1017/s0029665110001448.

Menon, V.P., and A.R. Sudheer (2007). "Antioxidant and Anti-Inflammatory Properties of Curcumin." In Aggarwal, B. B., Y. J. Surh, and S. Shishodia (eds) *The Molecular Targets and Therapeutic Uses of Curcumin in Health and Disease. Advances in Experimental Medicine and Biology,* vol. 595. Boston, MA: Springer. https://doi.org/10.1007/978-0-387-46401-5_3.

Mózsik, Gyula. "Capsaicin as New Orally Applicable Gastroprotective and Therapeutic Drug Alone or in Combination with Nonsteroidal Anti-Inflammatory Drugs in Healthy Human Subjects and in Patients." *Capsaicin as a Therapeutic Molecule* (2014): 209–58. https://doi.org/10.1007/978-3-0348-0828-6_9.

Ruggeri, Christine. "Cayenne Pepper Benefits Your Gut, Heart, and Beyond." Dr. Axe, May 27, 2018. https://draxe.com/nutrition/herbs/cayenne-pepper-benefits/.

Siddique, Ashik. "Za'atar Health Benefits: Middle Eastern Spice Blend Fights Microbes, May Boost Brain." *Medical Daily*, June 12, 2013. https://www.medicaldaily.com/zaatar-health-benefits-middle-eastern-spice-blend-fights-microbes-may-boost-brain-246726.

Silva, Nuno, et al. "Antimicrobial Activity of Essential Oils from Mediterranean Aromatic Plants against Several Foodborne and Spoilage Bacteria." *Food Science and Technology International* 19, no. 6 (February 26, 2013): 503–10. https://doi.org/10.1177/1082013212442198.

Tanaka, Takuji, Masahito Shnimizu, and Hisataka Moriwaki. "Cancer Chemoprevention by Carotenoids." *Molecules* 17, no. 3 (March 14, 2012): 3202–42. https://doi.org/10.3390/molecules17033202.

Truesdell, Delores D., Nancy R. Green, and Phyllis B. Acosta. "Vitamin B12 Activity in Miso and Tempeh." *Journal of Food Science* 52, no. 2 (March 1987): 493–94. https://doi.org/10.1111/j.1365-2621.1987.tb06650.x.

Anne, Melodie. "Which Is Better for You: Ground Turkey or Beef?" Livestrong.com. Accessed September 10, 2019. https://www.livestrong.com/article/496340-which-is-better-for-you-ground-turkey-or-beef/.

Chapter Six

Phillips, Katherine M., Amy S. Rasor, David M. Ruggio, and Karen R. Amanna. "Folate Content of Different Edible Portions of Vegetables and Fruits." Nutrition & Food Science. March 28, 2008. https://www.emerald.com/insight/content/doi/10.1108/00346650810863055/full/html.

Nordqvist, Christian. "All You Need to Know About Beta Carotene." Medical News Today. December 14, 2017. https://www.medicalnewstoday.com/articles/252758.php.

"Nutrition Facts for Pak-Choi (Bok Choy) (Cooked)." Myfooddata.com. Accessed August 26, 2019. https://tools.myfooddata.com/nutrition-facts.php?food=11117.

Ribeiro, Sônia Machado Rocha, et al. "Antioxidant in Mango (Mangifera Indica L.) Pulp." *Plant Foods for Human Nutrition* 62, no. 1 (2007): 13–17. https://doi.org/10.1007/s11130-006-0035-3.

"Basic Report: 11167, Corn, sweet, yellow, raw." USDA Food Composition Databases. April 2018. https://ndb.nal.usda.gov/ndb/foods/show/11167.

Bjarnadottir, Adda. "Beetroot 101: Nutrition Facts and Health Benefits." *Healthline*. March 8, 2019. https://www.healthline.com/nutrition/foods/beetroot#plant-compounds.

"Broccoli." SNAP Education Connection. Accessed August 26, 2019. https://snaped.fns.usda.gov/seasonal-produce-guide/broccoli.

Emerson, A. P. "Foods High in Fiber and Phytobezoar Formation." *Journal of Ethnopharmacology* 23, no. 2–3 (1988): 350–51. https://doi.org/10.1016/0378-8741(88)90063-3.

Ray, Ramesh C., and Didier Montet. *Microorganisms and Fermentation of Traditional Foods*. Boca Raton: CRC Press, Taylor & Francis Group, 2015.

"Cauliflower, Raw: Nutrition Facts & Calories." Nutrition Data. Accessed August 26, 2019. https://nutritiondata.self.com/facts/vegetables-an d-vegetable-products/239%.

O'Brien, Sharon. "15 Foods That Pack More Potassium Than a Banana." *Healthline.* July 26, 2018. https://www.healthline.com/nutrition /foods-loaded-with-potassium#section9.

USDA Food Composition Databases. Accessed August 26, 2019. https://ndb.nal.usda.gov/ndb/search.

Kubala, Jillian. "Swiss Chard: Nutrition, Benefits and How to Cook It." *Healthline.* December 4, 2018. https://www.healthline.com/nutrition /swiss-chard#heart-health.

Godman, Heidi. "Extra Protein Is a Decent Dietary Choice, but Don't Overdo It." *Harvard Health Blog*, May 1, 2013. https://www.health.harvard.edu/blog /extra-protein-is-a-decent-dietary-choice-but-dont-overdo-it-201305016145.

Paddon-Jones, et al. "Protein, Weight Management, and Satiety." *The American Journal of Clinical Nutrition* 87, no. 5 (January 2008). https://doi.org/10.1093/ajcn/87.5.1558s.

"Chickpea Pasta—High Protein, High Fiber, Gluten Free Pasta." Banza. Accessed August 26, 2019. https://www.eatbanza.com/.

"Refried and Other Canned Beans: Healthy or Not?" *Go Ask Alice!* Accessed August 26, 2019. https://goaskalice.columbia.edu/answered-questions /refried-and-other-canned-beans-healthy-or-not.

"Basic Report: 16015, Beans, black, mature seeds, cooked, boiled, without salt." USDA Food Composition Databases. April 2018. https://ndb.nal.usda.gov /ndb/foods/show/16015.

Dreher, Mark L., and Adrienne J. Davenport. "Hass Avocado Composition and Potential Health Effects." *Critical Reviews in Food Science and Nutrition* 53, no. 7 (2013): 738–50. https://doi.org/10.1080/10408398.2011.556759.

National Research Council (US) Committee on Diet and Health. "Fat-Soluble Vitamins." *Diet and Health: Implications for Reducing Chronic Disease Risk.* Washington, DC: National Academies Press, 1989. https://www.ncbi .nlm.nih.gov/books/NBK218749/.

"2013 International Year of Quinoa (IYQ2013)." Food and Agriculture Organi- zation of the United Nations. Accessed August 26, 2019. http://www.fao.org /quinoa-2013/what-is-quinoa/nutritional-value/en/.

McDonell, Kayla. "Brown vs. White Rice—Which Is Better for Your Health?" *Healthline*. August 31, 2016. https://www.healthline.com/nutrition /brown-vs-white-rice.

"Basic Report: 11457, Spinach, raw." USDA Food Composition Databases. April 2018. https://ndb.nal.usda.gov/ndb/foods/show/11457.

Nanasombat, Suree, and Pornpan Wimuttigosol. "Antimicrobial and Antioxidant Activity of Spice Essential Oils." *Food Science and Biotechnology* 20, no. 1 (2011): 45–53. https://doi.org/10.1007/s10068-011-0007-8.

"Healthy Reasons to Put Farro on Your Plate - Tufts University Health & Nutrition Letter Article." Health & Nutrition Letter. June 2015. https:// www.nutritionletter.tufts.edu/issues/11_6/current-articles/Healthy-Reason s-to-Put-Farro-on-Your-Plate_1727-1.html.

Chapter Seven

"Basic Report: 11007, Artichokes, (Globe or French), Raw." USDA Food Composition Databases. April 2018. https://ndb.nal.usda.gov/ndb/foods /show/11007.

"Basic Report: 12006, Seeds, Chia Seeds, Dried." USDA Food Composition Databases. April 2018. https://ndb.nal.usda.gov/ndb/foods/show/3610.

"Basic Report: 20137, Quinoa, Cooked." USDA Food Composition Databases. April 2018. https://ndb.nal.usda.gov/ndb/foods/show/305319.

Brown, Mary Jane. "Top 8 Health Benefits of Artichokes and Artichoke Extract." *Healthline*. January 16, 2019. https://www.healthline.com /nutrition/artichoke-benefits#section5.

Callaway, J. C. "Hempseed as a Nutritional Resource: An Overview." *Euphytica* 140, no. 1–2 (January 2004): 65–72. https://doi.org/10.1007 /s10681-004-4811-6.

"Full Report (All Nutrients): 45287121, PEPITAS PUMPKIN SEEDS KERNELS, UPC: 034952587371." USDA Food Composition Databases. July 2018. https://ndb.nal.usda.gov/ndb/foods/show/45287121.

Kirchhoff, R., et al. "Increase in Choleresis by Means of Artichoke Extract." *Phytomedicine* 1, no. 2 (September 1994): 107–15. https://doi .org/10.1016/s0944-7113(11)80027-9.

Morsy, Engy M. El, and Rehab Kamel. "Protective Effect of Artichoke Leaf Extract against Paracetamol-Induced Hepatotoxicity in Rats." *Pharmaceutical Biology* 53, no. 2 (February 2015): 167–73. https://doi.org/10.3109/13880209.2014.913066.

Sandoval-Oliveros, María R., and Octavio Paredes-López. "Isolation and Characterization of Proteins from Chia Seeds (Salvia Hispanica L.)." *Journal of Agricultural and Food Chemistry* 61, no. 1 (January 2013): 193–201. https://doi.org/10.1021/jf3034978.

Ullah, Rahman, et al. "Nutritional and Therapeutic Perspectives of Chia (Salvia Hispanica L.): A Review." *Journal of Food Science and Technology* 53, no. 4 (April 2016): 1750–58. https://doi.org/10.1007/s13197-015-1967-0.

RECIPE INDEX

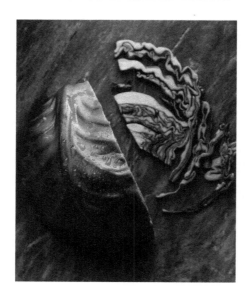

INDEX

T

V

ABOUT THE AUTHORS

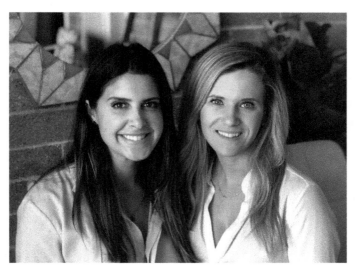

© April Murray/Leila Page

April Murray is a registered dietitian and nutritionist who practices and preaches that healthy food should taste good. Her passion for nutrition led her to found OC Nutrition Coaching. She earned her Bachelor of Science degree in clinical nutrition at University of California–Davis and completed her dietetic program at Stony Brook University in New York. April is a certified LEAP therapist and provides food sensitivity testing as well as nutrition coaching for thyroid health, weight loss, and other health conditions.

Leila Page is a registered dietitian and nutritionist who has a huge passion for nutrition. She earned her Bachelor of Science degree in food and nutrition science/dietetics at California State Polytechnic University and completed her dietetic program at University of Houston. During this journey she was led to OC Nutrition Coaching, working alongside April Murray. Her nutrition counseling specialties include weight loss, sports nutrition, healthy lifestyle, diabetes, pregnancy, cooking, and meal planning.